P9-DDN-841

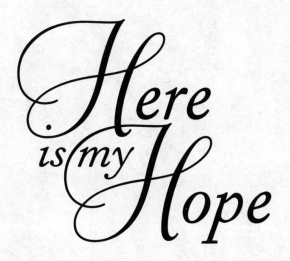

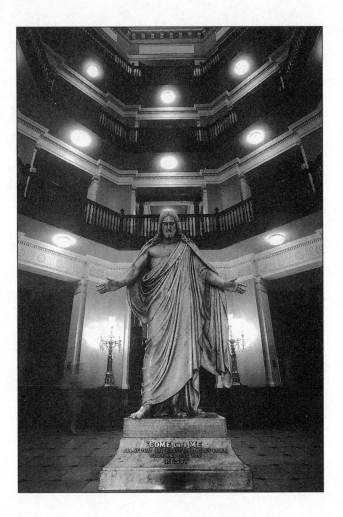

DOUBLEDAY
New York London Toronto Sydney Auckland

A Book of Healing and Prayer

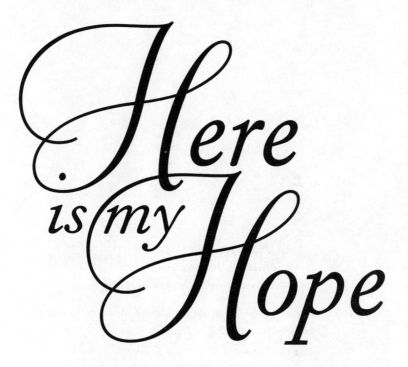

Here is my Hope

Inspirational Stories from The Johns Hopkins Hospital

RANDI HENDERSON
and RICHARD MAREK

PUBLISHED BY DOUBLEDAY
a division of Random House, Inc.
1540 Broadway, New York, New York 10036

DOUBLEDAY and the portrayal of an anchor with a dolphin are trademarks of
Doubleday, a division of Random House, Inc.

ISBN 0-385-50032-7
Copyright © 2001 by The Johns Hopkins Hospital
All Rights Reserved

"One Day at a Time": words and music by Marijohn Wilkin and
Kris Kristofferson, copyright © 1973, 1975 by
Buckhorn Music Publisher, Inc., BMI.
"He Smiled On Me": by Daniel S. Twohig; music by Geoffrey O'Hara,
copyright © 1939 by G. Schirmer, Inc.
Every effort has been made to contact the
above copyright holders for permission.

Book design by Fearn Cutler

Printed in the United States of America

$\mathscr{A}$cknowledgments

This book was inspired by an article in the *Baltimore Sun*, written by Diana Sugg. Diana's concept and her reporting were part of the foundation for our stories, and we thank her for her sensitive writing and sharp reporter's eye.

If Diana's article gave this work life, the efforts of Elaine Freeman and Judith Ehrlich gave it legs. Elaine, director of the Johns Hopkins Medicine Office of Communications and Public Affairs, and Judith, a literary agent with Linda Chester and Associates, both saw the potential for enlarging the scope of the newspaper article to encompass a series of detailed case studies. We thank Elaine and Judith for their vision and support for the project. We also extend our appreciation to Eric Major and his staff at Doubleday for their belief in this book and their help and encouragement.

Encouragement also came from leadership of The Johns Hopkins Hospital, including President Ronald R. Peterson, Vice President for Medical Affairs Beryl J. Rosenstein, M.D.; Vice President for Nursing and Patient Care Karen B. Haller, Ph.D.; and Director of Pastoral Care Stephen L. Mann. Drs. Rosenstein and Haller also served on a review committee with Drs. Patricia D. Fosarelli, Edward E. Wallach, and Benjamin S. Carson to assure the accuracy of medical information.

Dozens of other doctors and nurses, chaplains, secretaries, administrators, librarians, and other Hopkins staff members assisted in the research for this book. We thank them, with special appreciation to Gabriele Hourticolon of the Welch Medical Library and Nancy McCall of the Alan Mason Chesney Medical Archives.

Acknowledgments

Finally, we thank all of the people who opened their lives to our probing, who shared their deeply personal spiritual sensibilities, who relived painful and trying times with us. Their faith is truly an inspiration.

—Randi Henderson
—Richard Marek

Contents

INTRODUCTION
The Divine Healer

Thank You, kind Jesus, for my life again.

In the center of the main rotunda of The Johns Hopkins Hospital stands a towering statue of Christ. Arms outstretched in compassion, head bowed in beneficence, in His presence many find solace and peace. From dawn until late at night, patients in slippered feet and dragging IV poles, their families and loved ones, doctors, nurses, housekeepers and deliverymen, and visitors from all over the world reach to briefly touch the cool gray marble. Like those of the *Pietà* in Saint Peter's, the feet are worn smooth by those in need of His comfort.

Despite the traffic through the rotunda, the space around the statue is hushed. There is a feeling of reverence, a sense of being in a chapel. Frequently the pedestal on which Christ stands is piled with flowers. And often, a patient or relative or friend of a patient will leave, along with flowers, a written message: a prayer of hope, of consolation, of thanks.

Please God, let Wally's test results be favorable. Johns Hopkins is our only hope!

The statue is a copy of *Christus Consolator* or The Divine Healer by the Danish neoclassical sculptor Bertel Thorvaldsen. In the century it has stood in the Hopkins rotunda, it has come to represent not only the beliefs of Christianity but the compassion and humility honored in all religions. In this academic center, a leader in medical technology, it has evolved into a spiritual touchstone. To some, faith and science may seem unlikely partners. But most who come in contact with this marble figure find that it enhances the scientific healing offered at the hospital.

In fact, the story of how this presence came to this lobby is rooted in some very secular history. Johns Hopkins was a wealthy Quaker businessman who made his fortune first in the wholesale food business and later in banking. He endowed both the university and hospital in Baltimore that bear his name and had decidedly nonsectarian ideas about how these institutions should be oriented. His intention was that the hospital be a teaching and research facility with no religious affiliation. In the mid-nineteenth century, his type of thinking was radical—churches and hospitals had been linked since antiquity, and faith was seen as an integral part of the healing process. Hospitals were only beginning to be regarded as institutions with value for scientific merit alone.

Johns Hopkins died in 1873, and three years later the university established by his bequest was dedicated. In accordance with their perception of his wishes, the trustees he had handpicked to run the university marked its opening with a ceremony that contained no invocation, no benediction, no thanks to the Lord, and a keynote speaker known for his belief in evolution and other irreligious views. The dedication received local and national attention, and both the press and public expressed indignation at the exclusion of God from the ceremonies. "Many in the audience were shocked at the disrespect paid to religion," reported the *New York Observer*. In his memoirs, Daniel Coit Gilman, president of the university and hospital, spoke of the "black eye" the approach had earned the university and his desire to prevent it from happening again. At the dedication of the hospital in 1889, he specifically asked that a generous person donate a copy of the Thorvaldsen sculpture, which he had seen in his European travels, for the hospital lobby.

Such a statue, he predicted, would impart a powerful message: "With the outstretched hands of mercy, to remind each passerby—the physician and the nurse as they pursue their ministry of relief; the student as he begins his daily task; and the sufferer from injury or disease—that over all this institution rests the perpetual benediction of Christian charity, the constant spirit of good will to men."

William Wallace Spence—a Baltimore businessman, close friend of the late Johns Hopkins, and a pillar of the local Presbyterian church—responded to the request. Within two weeks, Gilman had written to the Danish embassy about the possibility of obtaining a copy of the statue and within another few months a deal was struck for a marble replica for the sum of twenty thousand Danish crowns—about $5,360. In November 1894 the statue's location was set when the Board of Trustees unanimously adopted a resolution to place it "immediately under the Dome in the main hall of [the] Administration Building."

It took nearly seven years for the commission to be executed. The Divine Healer, ten and a half feet tall and weighing six tons, carved out of a single block of marble, arrived in the Baltimore Harbor in the autumn of 1896 and was loaded onto a large wooden cart. Four horses pulled the cart up Broadway from the docks, past the front door of the hospital and around to the north entrance. It was unloaded there, pushed down the short corridor, and raised up on the pedestal, which had been constructed locally, to its permanent resting place directly under the dome.

At the dedication of the statue on October 14, 1896, Spence explained his motivation for his gift to the hospital:

To every weary sufferer entering these doors the first object presented to him is this benign gracious figure looking down upon him with pitying eyes and outstretched arms, and as it

were saying to him, "Come unto Me and I will give you rest."
I thought it might help to comfort some sad and weary one
and lead his heart and thoughts up to the everlasting Divine
Healer, and Who alone could give that rest.

More than eight hundred people watched Spence's four-year-old
great-granddaughter pull the string that released the muslin cloth covering the statue. These included patients gathered on the staircase and
nurses and doctors looking down from the upper tiers. Then, as now,
those seeing the statue for the first time were awestruck. The trustees'
account of the ceremony noted that when the statue was unveiled, "the
effect upon the audience of this presence was so impressive that they
were awed into silent admiration, rather than moved to applause."

Another speaker, William Dixon, president of the Board of
Trustees, spoke with prescience of the role this statue would play in
the future. "Not only are the outstretched hands of this *Christus Consolator* held out to this company, this community, and the people of
this age," he said, "but they will remain extended to tens of thousands of the generations yet to come."

A century later . . .

Dixon was correct. The hope, the consolation, and the love symbol-
ized by The Divine Healer have continued for generations. But today
the statue represents another, modern dimension. For even as our
medicine has come to rely more and more on technological innovation and the wonders of science, doctors have increasingly become
aware of the role of spirituality in the healing process. Even as the
twentieth century put a wall between science and spirituality, the
clear direction of the twenty-first century is to breach that wall and
unite the two disciplines.

Mind, body, and emotion, we now recognize, are inextricably
linked. Eastern medicine has long understood the importance of spir-

ituality as a facet of healing. Many books describe the correlation of psychological stress and physical disease. Hospitals are hiring more chaplains. Physicians are going back to school to be trained as ministers. Prayer groups are becoming permanent fixtures in some intensive care units. Nationally, in 1994, only three medical schools taught courses that included religion and spirituality. By 1999, the number had increased to sixty, nearly one half of all medical schools. At The Johns Hopkins Hospital, a chaplain has become a daily presence in all seven intensive care units and the adult and pediatric emergency rooms, and the medical school offers a course on medicine and religion.

Studies show that most people want religion or spirituality in their lives. And their doctors want it too. Surveys have found that nearly 80 percent of Americans think that the power of God or prayer can improve health and lead to healing. Physicians treating terminal patients report that nearly 70 percent of patients request spiritual counseling or referral. And a study of family physicians found that 79 percent of the doctors categorized themselves as having a strong religious or spiritual orientation. At Hopkins, many physicians rub the toe of Jesus as they pass—often going out of their way to do so, since the Broadway rotunda is no longer the main lobby and crossroads of the hospital.

Religion and spirituality have also attracted scrutiny in a growing body of scientific investigation in diverse areas. A 1998 Hopkins study by psychiatrist Peter Rabins found that when caretakers of people with Alzheimer's disease had emotional support, including religious faith, they were better able to handle difficult tasks and emotional stresses, which sometimes translated to a delay in the need to institutionalize family members with Alzheimer's. Hopkins neurologist Michael Williams is teaching physicians to help families make decisions for patients in intensive care, with the identification of spiritual needs as an important facet of this work.

In medical centers around the country and the world, scientists are testing the role of faith and prayer against a variety of diseases and conditions—high blood pressure, AIDS, heart disease, cancer, gastrointestinal diseases, mental illness, and others. Hundreds of studies can now be found in the medical literature. In an attempt to quantify the role of religion and spirituality in healing, scientists at the University of Florida have developed an assessment tool, the Spiritual Involvement and Beliefs Scale, and initial testing indicates good reliability and validity. This and similar instruments are likely to have an increasing role in scientific study. Indeed, few today would argue the role of faith and religion in the healing process. The following list is just a sample of the work that has been done:

~ A study at Duke University of an elderly population found that people who attended religious services at least once a week and prayed or studied the Bible daily had lower blood pressure than those with less frequent religious activities.

~ Another blood pressure study followed a group of nuns and a group of lay women over thirty years. In that period, the blood pressure of the nuns remained steady, while that of the lay women increased, as might be expected with aging. The lay women also had more heart and cardiovascular problems.

~ Another Duke study found that people who were unaffiliated with a religious community had longer hospital stays than those with a religious affiliation. The contrast was striking—the hospital stays of those with religious affiliations averaged eleven days, compared to twenty-five days for the others.

~ A study of nearly two thousand elderly people in North Carolina found that churchgoers had stronger immune systems than nonchurchgoers. Those who attended church at least weekly were half as likely as the nonattendees to have elevated levels of interleukin 6, which has been associated with tumor growth and autoimmune disease.

~ Studies of behavior and public health also point to the healing potential of faith and prayer. Two recent studies (December 1998) emphasize that religious involvement may discourage use of tobacco and abuse of alcohol and other drugs, behaviors that are clearly related to increased health risks.

~ At the University of California–Berkeley, over a twenty-eight-year period, studies found the risk of dying prematurely from grave illness was almost 25 percent less (35 percent for women) for people who attend religious services frequently.

~ A study of more than ninety thousand people in western Maryland found that regular churchgoers had lower death rates from coronary artery disease (50 percent reduction), emphysema (56 percent), cirrhosis (74 percent), and suicide (53 percent).

~ Dartmouth researchers found that patients are twelve times more likely to survive open heart surgery if they have religious faith and social support.

~ A twenty-eight-year study of five thousand Californians found that women who went to religious worship services at least once a week had lifespans averaging seven years longer than non-worshipers.

~ A double-blind randomized study of advanced AIDS patients at the California Pacific Medical Center found that distant praying (praying from afar, without subjects knowing they are being prayed for) resulted in significantly fewer AIDS-related illnesses, less severe illnesses, fewer and shorter hospitalizations, and improved mood in the patients who were the subject of the distant prayers.

~ A double-blind study of 393 cardiac patients in San Francisco found that those who were the subjects of prayer by home prayer groups, even though they did not know they were being prayed for, did significantly better than those who were not prayed for.

While the outcomes of these studies almost always point to a beneficial effect from prayer and spirituality, researchers agree that a broader and more systematic study of this phenomenon is necessary to understand how and why it works and how it can be applied to the practice of modern medicine. But even as studies continue and proliferate, a different kind of work goes on under the Hopkins dome, where faith and science intersect.

Introduction

Dear Lord, thank You for not taking Whitney, thank You for her good kidney report. And I beg and pray of You, let the swelling in her brain be gone in tomorrow's CT scan.

In the century since The Divine Healer came to Hopkins, the physical plant has grown and shifted and the main entrance is now several buildings and corridors away, at the opposite side of the hospital. Perhaps Johns Hopkins, the man, would have preferred it this way. Many patients and visitors come and go without seeing The Divine Healer. But many others are told of the commanding statue and find themselves at his feet, offering their prayers. And it is still the place where people meet for lunch, for Christmas caroling, for other get-togethers—there is no mistaking the location.

Most people, when told that the statue stands ten and a half feet tall, are surprised. They think it is at least twice that height. The optical illusion is a result of several factors—the pedestal, which adds several feet to the height; the flowing lines of the robes; the dome above it, arching skyward. And, for many, the actual physical height is augmented by the spiritual and emotional impact of *Christus Consolator,* Christ the Consoler.

Our aim in *Here Is My Hope* is to be of inspirational help in the healing process—healing not only of the sick themselves, but of their loved ones when confronted with loss or the emotional anguish of serious illness. Our aim is to show inspiration in action—how others' lives have been changed and helped by the power of faith and the power of prayer.

You are about to meet a variety of men, women, and children, their lives interrupted by illness, their suffering eased by the combination of technology and prayer. Their stories will touch your heart and stir your faith. Among them:

~ A child with intractable seizures prays he will not need to undergo a hemispherectomy, the extreme procedure of removing half the brain perfected at Hopkins.

~ A young couple struggles with the pain of their grief as their premature twins tenuously cling to life in the neonatal intensive care unit.

~ A Catholic pediatrician learns that medical training is not enough when she begins to work with inner city children and their many health problems.

~ An eight-year-old boy, one of only a handful of children in the world to be struck with pancreatic cancer, writes his own prayer—not for himself, but for others.

~ An internationally known cardiac surgeon holds his own father's heart in his hand and wills it to resume beating.

These and five other stories are connected by a single theme—the power of faith and the representation of that power in The Divine Healer. The stories are about individual human beings. But their themes are ecumenical and faith itself is universal. In ten stories we can see the stories of ten million, all those in need of spiritual sustenance in times of crisis or despair.

We've broken the book into three sections—Hope, Consolation, and Thanks. But really the book is seamless, for The Divine Healer is present in each story, no matter the specific kind of faith involved. Each of the chapters opens and closes with prayer. We hope that by reading the stories you find inspiration for your own life, your own travails, your own feelings of hope and hopelessness, despair and thanksgiving. If the book gives you strength and insight, if it convinces you that spiritual forces can work in conjunction with technology and medicine—and in some cases heal even when medicine fails—if in its stories of others it illuminates your own path, then it will have achieved its purpose.

Thank You, Lord, for my Christmas present—my life. Amen.

Part One

HOPE

GRAYSON GILBERT
Reaching Up

*Dear Lord, Thank You for our kingdom, from
GraFson.*

—NOVEMBER 2, 1998

On a crisp fall afternoon, eight-year-old Grayson Gilbert pauses
to leave a note at the base of the Christ statue. Despite his age, he is
no stranger to these halls, and has left notes at the foot of The
Divine Healer before. He's at Hopkins for a six-month checkup,
more than two years after a bout with pancreatic cancer, a disease
that children almost never get and, if they do, rarely survive. Three
years ago, no one would have dared predict a healthy future for
Grayson. Today everyone he has seen—the oncologist, the surgeon,
the endocrinologist, the radiologist, all the nurses and techs—have
been smilingly delighted with his good health. You can't *not* smile at
this sweet, sunny, engaging boy. He bounds into the rotunda, a burst
of energy, takes a lap around Jesus, and jumps up under the outstretched arm, going for a high five. He can't quite reach. In a way,
though, he certainly has.

*Dear Jesus, This is Grayson. If You could just heal the other kids,
please. Thank You very much.*

—MAY 8, 1996

When he wrote this note, Grayson Gilbert was only six but knew all too well there were sick kids who needed healing. He had been through an ordeal himself. There had been weeks of hospitalization, a disruption from his normal home life with his parents and big brother, Wesley, and the new baby, Harrison. Surgery, chemotherapy, more surgery, still more surgery, more chemo, radiation—his young mind couldn't quite sort it out: the rarity and deadliness of the disease he'd had, the fact that the challenge to his health was far from over. But on this hopeful May morning, healed from surgery and leaving the hospital after a round of chemotherapy, he knew he felt well and there were other children who were not so fortunate. So his prayers were for them.

And somehow, this blue-eyed, fair-haired (but now bald) child connected his recovery—and the hopes for recovery of the other sick children he had met—with this statue and the faith it embodied. From the time of his first visits to The Johns Hopkins Hospital months before, he and his parents had been struck by the power of the marble figure in the Broadway lobby. It made Grayson feel he was cared for. Someone who could do more for him, even, than his parents and the doctors. "Mommy, before I go to surgery, can we make a note to Jesus?" he asked before his operation in February. Now he was leaving the hospital after a round of chemo, and he wanted to deposit another note. This prayer was not for himself. It was for those still on the cancer floor of the Children's Center, the kids who had become his friends and support system, the kids who weren't yet well enough to go home and maybe never would be.

For Grayson, the road to Johns Hopkins and the Jesus statue began with dull pain that wouldn't go away, increasing lethargy that alarmed his parents, and, finally, a diagnosis that was presented almost as a death sentence.

It was summer 1995 when the first hints of trouble came. Stephen and Jodie Gilbert were busy with the baby, born August 22. Gradually they became aware that Grayson, normally what his mother described as a "run-around" kid, wasn't as energetic as usual. He was keeping to himself, withdrawn, definitely not his customary talkative self. His appetite had practically disappeared; he would eat a few bites and say he was full. *This isn't Grayson,* Jodie and Steve thought, and even his friends noticed something different. But there were plenty of relatively benign possible explanations for his behavior. *Maybe he's afraid of starting kindergarten,* Jodie thought. *Maybe it's the fear of riding the school bus. Maybe he's in the middle of a growth spurt. Maybe it's just a reaction to the new baby.* A medical exam by the family doctor in August found no apparent problems.

Grayson started kindergarten at Stoneleigh Elementary School, a few blocks from his home in Towson, a suburb just north of Baltimore. A couple of weeks into the school year, his parents had a conference with the guidance counselor who said Grayson appeared fine but seemed to be keeping to himself. It was uncharacteristic and Jodie and Steve were concerned. They asked the counselor and Grayson's teacher to keep close watch on the five-year-old. After two weeks of observation, the counselor said she suspected the boy had some sort of physical problem.

Indeed, Steve and Jodie were noticing new physical signs. More and more, Grayson would assume an unusual posture, bending his right arm, holding it behind his back with his left hand grasping the right arm at the elbow. "Why do you keep doing that, sweetie?" Jodie asked, and he answered with a shrug. "It's just how I feel comfortable." Outside with his friends, he squatted and watched them play, rarely joining in, holding the arm behind his back. Sometimes he just lay down in the driveway and said he was tired. Middle-of-the-night headaches woke him up and he would lie in pain, not wanting to bother his parents again. And he was eating less and less, losing weight but always complaining of feeling full.

One evening in October, Jodie stood Grayson before her and did a head-to-toe examination of his body, an inch-by-inch palpation of her son's slight frame, seeking through the acute sensitivity of a mother's hands anything that might be causing the boy's symptoms. When she reached his belly, it felt hard. *What is going on here?* she asked herself in alarm, taking care to hide her fears from Grayson. *This can't be right.*

The next day was a Saturday, but Grayson's pediatrician said he would see him. The doctor agreed there was a mass of some sort in Grayson's abdomen and told Jodie that Grayson should see a general surgeon and get a sonogram as soon as possible. Monday morning found Jodie and Grayson at a nearby community hospital, where a sonogram confirmed an abnormality. Jodie, sensing that something serious was happening, had suggested that Steve take the other two boys to a toy store to divert them. The surgeon told Jodie that further diagnosis and treatment were probably beyond the capabilities of this small facility, and Grayson should go to Johns Hopkins for evaluation. Immediately.

Bewildered and frightened, Jodie and Steve met at home. They didn't even know how to get to Hopkins, in downtown Baltimore. While Steve called for directions, Jodie threw together an overnight bag for Grayson—pajamas, a change of clothes, a book about Batman, with whom he was enthralled. Her instincts were screaming, *This is bad, this is real bad.* With all three boys, Harrison nursing at her breast, they piled into the car. Steve and Jodie tried to protect Grayson from the dread they were feeling, yet the drive to Hopkins was filled with tense silence. Formless prayers were running through their heads. *Oh God, please God . . .* the prayers didn't go much further than that as they were loath to crystalize their fears into words or thought. *Oh God, please God . . .*

The Hopkins pediatric emergency room was quiet, in a dinnertime lull when the Gilberts arrived at about five-thirty P.M., and they didn't have to wait long to be seen. The next couple of hours were filled with a succession of doctors, their expressions solemn, examining Grayson's belly, asking him how he felt, where it hurt, getting all the background they could. Allen Chen, the pediatric oncologist on call, examined Grayson alone, without his parents around, and was impressed with how articulate the little boy was, how well he was able to describe his symptoms. But he didn't like the feel of Grayson's belly and thought it was unlikely they were dealing with anything but a malignancy.

Finally Eric Strauch, a young pediatric surgery fellow, beckoned Steve and Jodie out of the waiting area, sat them down in a small cubicle, and put words to their fears. "There is definitely a mass, and it is probably cancerous," he told them gravely, knowing from the hard, firm feel of the mass that there was no point in offering false hope. "We need to do another CAT scan to find out more about it, how extensive it is, and Grayson will have to be admitted to the hospital."

Jodie gasped, wanting to know more but having trouble comprehending what she was hearing. Steve felt thrown back, as though he'd been hit with a cannonball. This was the exact news he'd been praying *not* to hear for the past three days. He broke down in tears. Jodie didn't cry. She understood she had to be stronger than she'd ever been, fought through the fog that threatened to envelop her, and she reached inward for the steel core of faith she knew she needed to keep her family going.

It was another two hours before Grayson got into the CAT scan. From the little cubicle where they waited, Jodie and Steve started calling family: Steve's parents, his brother and sister, Jodie's sister. By ten P.M., when Grayson was finally taken down to radiology for the scan, a half-dozen family members had gathered. Steve's brother and his wife took Wesley and Harrison home for the night. *How many nights will it be?* everyone wondered. This was just the beginning.

Grayson didn't think he was sick enough to be in the hospital. None of this hurt very much and everyone was nice, but he didn't want to stay. He was angry, especially at his mother, who had started all this, rushing him to the doctor on a weekend. He turned a stony face to Jodie and would only talk to Steve.

From the CAT scan, Grayson was taken to a room on the eighth floor of the Children's Center, 8E, the oncology unit for young children. Surgery was scheduled for the next morning. The doctors were going to spend some time examining the scans, and didn't have any more information for Steve and Jodie. "Is this a surgery he'll survive?" Steve asked Strauch, choking out the question, barely able to give words to his worst fears. "We don't know," the doctor answered gently. "We'll do our best." He told the numb couple to try to get some sleep in the reclining chairs in Grayson's room. They arranged the chairs at the corner of the bed, so they could clutch hands across the bed and both still have physical contact with Grayson. He looked so small in the hospital bed, almost like a baby again. Steve rubbed his back, Jodie put her head next to her son's shiny blond one. They spent the night in a tight threesome, Grayson sleeping for a while, his parents hardly at all. Steve and Jodie barely spoke. What was there to say?

In the morning, they met Walter Pegoli, the pediatric surgeon who would operate on Grayson, with Strauch assisting. Pegoli was compassionate and thorough, but it wouldn't be until after the surgery that he could really tell them what was going on in Grayson's abdomen. Jodie and Steve assumed that he would be cutting out the tumor, but Pegoli and Strauch knew that much of what they would be doing would be exploratory. Even with the CAT scan, they couldn't tell exactly where the tumor was, where it originated, what organs or blood vessels might be involved. Pegoli told Jodie and Steve that the surgery might be very complicated and could take a long time, maybe as long as eight hours.

One parent could accompany Grayson into the operating room, and he chose his father. He was still acting angry with Jodie for starting all this, wouldn't talk to her or meet her eye. She went back and forth between thinking it was funny and feeling hurt. *At least he's showing emotion,* she thought. *He's just being a kid.*

Even Pegoli didn't anticipate how complicated the surgery would be. The procedure took five and one-half hours. The dark firm malignant mass, visually distinct from the healthy tissue and organs in Grayson's abdomen, was squeezing off major blood vessels. To compensate, his body had created a collateral network of vessels that kept blood flowing to his organs. But the tumor was intertwined with everything, an overshadowing presence. It would have to be shrunk before it could safely come out. The doctors excised a golf-ball-size sample and closed Grayson up again.

And whithersoever He entered, into villages, or cities, or country, they laid the sick in the streets and besought Him that they might touch if it were but the border of His garment: and as many as touched Him were made whole.

—MARK 6:56

During the long wait, family members again gathered for support and prayer. As they clustered in a corner of the waiting room and held hands, Steve's father, one of the dedicated churchgoers in the group, reassured everyone with prayers of hope, such as the comforting description of healing from Mark. Jodie and Steve heard a few times from the patient representative during the surgery: that Grayson was holding his own, that he had lost some blood and needed transfusion, that they would have to wait for the surgeon to tell them what he had done. Wesley and Harrison were with their aunt, not at the hospital, and all day long Jodie felt that her breasts were bursting and the front of her blouse was soaked with the milk that Harrison wasn't there to take.

Finally, Pegoli was there, still in his green scrubs, mask dangling around his neck. He took Jodie and Steve aside to explain what had happened—and what hadn't. "This is a very serious situation," he told them, not downplaying anything. "We had to bail out because if we had kept on going, he might have died. We were only able to do a biopsy because the tumor was so large. If we had tried to take it out now, it would have been extremely life threatening."

Jodie and Steve couldn't believe what they were hearing. Whatever their son had in his belly, it was something rarely seen. Pegoli had to wait for the pathology report to be positive of what it was. But he thought they were looking at a pancreatoblastoma, a malignant tumor growing out of Grayson's pancreas, the organ behind the stomach that produces insulin and digestive hormones and is essential for life. Grayson's tumor was the size of a large grapefruit. It was wound around his duodenum, the upper part of the small intestine, and was involved with his aorta and vena cava, the body's primary blood vessels. It had wrapped around his portal vein, coming out from the liver, and the superior mesenteric artery and vein, which take blood to and from the mesentery, the thick band of tissue that encases the organs of the abdomen.

"Here's the deal, here's what we have to do," Pegoli said. He needed to do some research to find out more about pancreatic tumors in children. The oncologist had to find out which drugs showed the most promise against this type of tumor. It would take about two weeks for Grayson to recover sufficiently from surgery to begin chemotherapy. Then he would be started on a regimen that, hopefully, would shrink the tumor to an operable size. That would take months longer. Then they would operate and take out the tumor. After that, Grayson might need radiation and more chemotherapy.

Pancreatic cancer is one of the least curable cancers. In children, it is particularly difficult to predict its course because it is seen so rarely. Pegoli made that sound like almost good news to the Gilberts—those horrible survival rates didn't have to apply to Grayson. Steve and Jodie felt reassured about the steps that had been laid out.

There was a plan, the doctors were on top of this. Jodie thought that Pegoli's dark brown eyes were reassuring and caring. They felt that Grayson was in good hands.

When Walt Pegoli and Allen Chen set out to research pancreatic cancer in children, they didn't find much. Reports about pancreatic cancer in general are not very heartening. Of the 27,000 Americans who get this type of cancer each year, only 25 percent survive for a year. "Cancer of the . . . pancreas is rarely curable," begins a report for physicians from the National Cancer Institute. The five-year survival rate is a dismal 4 percent.

But what did this mean for Grayson? Eighty percent of cases are in people over the age of sixty. The National Cancer Database, an electronic registry cosponsored by the American Cancer Society and the American College of Surgeons didn't even have a category for childhood pancreatic cancer—it lumped all patients under the age of fifty in a single group. Most doctors, even pediatric surgeons in large medical centers, have never seen pancreatic cancer in a child. Pegoli had seen one previous case.

As they dug further, the doctors started finding some more encouraging accounts. There was a smattering of reports on pancreatoblastomas in children from around the world, and many of these children seemed to be doing well. Doctors at Memorial Sloan-Kettering Cancer Center in New York followed six children with pancreatoblastomas and five of them were alive, surviving from twenty-two months to twenty-two years. Doctors in Indiana reported the case of a ten-year-old who was alive and disease free six years after surgery. From Italy, there was news of a girl who was operated on for a pancreatoblastoma when she was six and four years later was doing well.

Several of the reports mentioned success with chemotherapy. Doctors from Japan and France had good results shrinking tumors with chemotherapy before operating, just what the doctors were proposing for Grayson. Everyone with any experience with the disease seemed to be urging aggressive surgery. That would come for Grayson, but now the surgeons turned the case over to the oncologists who would try to shrink the tumor.

~

It took seventeen days for Grayson and the doctors to be ready to begin chemo. Recovering from surgery, he was given midazolam (Versed), a muscle relaxant that kept him from fighting the ventilator, a frequent problem with children in critical care. Versed has the added property of causing amnesia, so Grayson didn't remember much about those few blurry days. Soon he was up and about, though, exploring the halls. The staff and other patients and parents called him Speedy, for the little Speedy Gonzales toy he carried around.

The drugs decided upon for Grayson were doxorubicin (Adriamycin) and cisplatin, two aggressive chemotherapy drugs with a wide range of possible side effects, from alopecia (hair loss) to heart failure to deafness. Baldness didn't bother Grayson—he would playfully compare his bald head to Harrison's, who didn't grow hair until after his first birthday. And modern chemotherapy, with many drugs to counter the toxic side effects of the anticancer weapons, is no longer the sentence of misery it once was. It was no fun, but Grayson weathered it well. By now he was used to having his blood drawn, which made him feel sort of scared and sort of cool at the same time. He got to lie around a lot and watch movies, and that wasn't so bad. Grayson stayed in the hospital the entire time: the seventeen days while he recovered and the doctors plotted their course, and then another week when he was actually getting the chemo.

He didn't know what it meant to have cancer, or even what cancer was, but he could tell it was bad from the way his parents and everyone else acted. The person who helped him most was Lauren

McCarthy, his first roommate. A thirteen-year-old girl from southern Maryland, she had bone cancer in her leg and was getting chemotherapy. Steve and Jodie saw the spirited gleam of life in her eyes as she introduced herself and told Grayson about cancer and chemo and what this was all about. "Chemo sucks," she said, "but you know, we're strong. We're going to make it." She was full of smiles and laughter and made Grayson feel strong. She told him about things he could do in the hospital—the arts and crafts room soon became a favorite. On Halloween, she took him there for a pumpkin-carving contest and he won second place.

Steve felt a psychological and emotional boost from Lauren's cheerful, practical, positive outlook. As the days went by, he saw another side of her, the tears that weren't very far below the surface, the appreciation she had for the fact that she was in a fight for her life. He spent as much time as he could at the hospital, stepping back from the real estate appraising business he had with his father. Not that he could really afford to—Jodie was a full-time stay-at-home mom and they pretty much lived from paycheck to paycheck. If he wasn't working, there wasn't going to be any income coming in, but that seemed like a minor worry right now. Somehow they'd manage. At least they had health insurance to cover most of Grayson's medical costs.

Steve spent nights in the room with Grayson while Jodie left the hospital in the evening to pick up Harrison and Wesley from the friend or neighbor or relative who was helping for the day. She spent the nights with them at home, trying to give them some semblance of normalcy. Harrison, of course, was too young for any of this to have an emotional impact, but Wesley was ten and understood plenty. Hearing that his little brother had cancer was very frightening, especially since his parents couldn't hide how scared they were. Wesley struggled to understand why Grayson had gotten cancer—he didn't know of anyone else in his family who had ever had it. When he visited him in the hospital, Grayson didn't seem that bad, but Wesley suddenly became aware of a world he'd never seen before, a world of suffering and sorrow. He heard parents crying, he heard kids moaning and sometimes screaming because something hurt. The observations and experiences left their mark—Wesley would never again be quite the innocent child he once had been.

In those weeks at the hospital, Steve felt he was fighting his way through a whirlwind, trying to figure out what this meant for all of their lives. *My life has definitely changed,* he thought, *but is this going to be a good or a bad story?* He pulled himself back from an image that kept creeping in—himself at a cemetery burying Grayson. Better to visualize happy endings. He made it his mission to meet everyone else on the floor, patients and parents. This was facilitated when his brother-in-law came in one day with a huge tub of bubblegum for Grayson. Steve went from room to room, offering the gum to all, gratified by the smiles and positive responses he got from nearly everyone. But he wasn't prepared for the disease toll he saw, the evidence of illness that was impossible to mask with smiles. Kids hooked up to tubes, many of them emaciated and weak, sometimes crying, some of them clearly near death—it was a sobering journey but Steve kept on going. "My son Grayson is in room 805 and they don't give him much of a chance of living," he told the other patients and their parents. "But he's going to beat it. And he got this big thing of gum we want to share with you."

Steve became actively involved with Grayson's care, learning to give injections, monitoring the tubes, providing some relief for the overworked nurses. As the hospitalization stretched on, he'd see a lost, stricken look on the faces of parents with kids just coming into the hospital, the look he knew he'd had himself, and he went out of his way to comfort people. Suddenly he was a *de facto* parent counselor for the floor, teaching the moms and dads who stayed with their kids the most comfortable way to turn the reclining chair in the room into a bed, sharing other practical tips and advice. The hospital has a way of shutting out the world, and for those weeks Steve's total energy was centered on CMSC–8E, with the tightest focus on his son but with plenty of waves emanating outward to the rest of the unit.

Grayson finally went home in November after nearly four weeks in the hospital, the last week devoted to his first round of chemo. This was just the beginning for chemo, and as a reminder he had a port in his chest, a semipermanent entryway for the IV needle. He would be home for three weeks, and then back in the hospital for another week of chemo. Home for three weeks, hospital again for one week. No one could say exactly how long this routine would continue. The tumor would be monitored with CAT scans and the doctors would decide when it was time to operate.

You can get used to anything, Jodie thought sometimes in those unsettling months when, as soon as she got used to one routine, she began another. It was a different kind of Thanksgiving, with blessings that seemed mixed at best; a different kind of Christmas, with the overhanging thought—what will next Christmas be like? But at least they were all together and managing to make it from one day to the next.

One day early in the new year, while Grayson was in the hospital for chemo, they met with the doctors to go over the proposed surgery. After the meeting, Steve grabbed her hand and Grayson's and said, "There's something you have to see." He led them to the Children's Center elevator and down to the first floor, and through the busy corridors that connect the various wings and buildings of the hospital. He knew Jodie was fighting depression, and he had stumbled upon the Christ statue one day in his travels around the hospital. Jodie hadn't seen it yet.

Sometimes Jodie was overwhelmed with despair. Even before Grayson had become sick, she had been going through some bad times, wondering why life had to be so difficult, questioning her faith, which had always been strong, if not totally conventional. She felt surrounded by death and disease, weighed down by continuing sorrow. Her mother had died four years ago. Before she conceived Harrison, she'd had an ectopic pregnancy and was mourning her lost baby, and paying an additional toll with painful complications from the surgery to her ruptured fallopian tube. She was nursing her father through Alzheimer's disease and he was doing poorly. *Everything is so hopeless,* she kept thinking, *where is my hope?*

Where is my hope? Jodie felt she'd lost the capacity for it. And now her boy was in and out of the hospital and doctors talked about less than 10 percent survival rates. *Where is my hope?* The thought kept going through her mind, she couldn't shake it. But when Steve led her into the rotunda in the old lobby, as she came around the huge staircase and caught her first glimpse of The Divine Healer, she suddenly felt she had an answer to her question.

Here is my hope, Jodie thought, and hope and faith and reassurance seemed to flow through her, a physical feeling, a sensation of warmth and comfort. She was awed by the figure, the beauty of the carving, the shadows, the lifelike aspect. It was not anything she had expected to see in this scientific institution. She felt transfixed.

It was morning, about ten A.M., and the lobby was filled with the usual bustle of hospital traffic. But all the activity faded into the background and Jodie felt it was just she and Jesus standing there. She stopped in her tracks and gazed at the statue and the reflected light in the rotunda. *Here is my hope.* She had not thought such comfort was possible. *My last hope.* She felt all her faith pour out of her into the statue and then flow back into her. Suddenly, a happy outcome seemed possible. She knelt and prayed. *Please Jesus, please help Grayson be a survivor.*

The doctors were encouraged by what they were seeing—the tumor was shrinking. In mid-February, while Grayson was in the hospital for another chemo treatment, Drs. Pegoli, Strauch, Chen, and Dome, the pediatric oncology fellow, called Jodie and Steve into an office where Grayson's scans from October and February, the first and the last, were mounted on a viewer. The tumor had shrunk from the size of a grapefruit to the size of a plum. It was time to take it out.

Here, finally, was hope to fill both Jodie's and Steve's hearts. From the meeting with the doctors, they paid a visit with their son to The Divine Healer. Someone else had left a single rose at Jesus' foot. Grayson slid a note under the flower:

Dear Jesus, please help the doctors and the caped crusader attack the bad guys in my tummy. Our thoughts and prayers are with You. Love, Grayson and Mom.

The surgery was scheduled for the next day, February 22, 1996. Grayson chose the clothes he would wear to the hospital—Batman cape, Batman mask, Batman socks, Batman underwear. The nurses let him keep the underwear on when he changed to his hospital gown. A local television station interviewed him for a feature, since this was such a rare cancer. Grayson was unconcernedly playing with his Fisher Price Little People on the playroom floor while the reporter rattled off the bleak survival statistics. Jodie was proud of how brave he was—after all he'd been through, he was still acting like a normal little boy. She'd been afraid that he would cry, and set off her and Steve, but everyone remained dry-eyed for the moment. A little while later, though, when Steve walked him into the operating room, grasping his hand, Grayson looked up and said, "Dad, it's going to be okay." Steve couldn't keep back the tears then, as he handed Grayson over to the anesthesiologist.

The gathered family knew they would again have a long wait—Pegoli had said that the operation would last eight hours or more, a tedious surgery with many potential complications. The surgeons knew as soon as they were inside Grayson's abdomen that they had hours of daunting work ahead of them. The shrunken tumor was coming from the pancreas but it was hard to pinpoint its original source. A frozen section biopsied during surgery confirmed that it was growing out of the head of the pancreas. The surgeons did a Whipple procedure, a pancreaticoduodenectomy that has been the standard of care for pancreatic cancer for decades. This operation removes the head of the pancreas but preserves enough of the organ to continue producing insulin. It also takes out sections of small intestine, gallbladder, bile duct, and pancreas and then reconnects the gastrointestinal tract so the patient can eat and digest normally. The Whipple has been refined by Hopkins surgeons who have much higher survival rates than national averages—but almost exclusively on adult patients.

In Grayson, one of the biggest challenges was the web of collateral blood vessels that had grown around the tumor. They had to be tied off to get to the tumor. The tumor and the chemotherapy had scarred and obstructed the portal vein, which drains blood from the small bowel to the liver. With the collateral vessels tied off, the bowel started to swell dangerously.

Even shrunken as it was, the tumor was still attached in many places, and the surgery involved a tremendous amount of laborious resection. After about five hours, the patient representative told Steve and Jodie that Grayson had lost a lot of blood; four replacement units had already been used. An hour later Strauch came to talk to them. He did not sound optimistic. "It's taking such a long time, we're thinking of stopping where we are and closing him up without getting it all out," he said. A half hour later Paul Colombani, chief of pediatric surgery, who was also in the operating room, came to talk to them. "Dr. Pegoli is taking heroic measures," he said, "but it might be a good idea if you called your clergyman."

The Gilberts already had two clergypeople waiting with them, and the medical reports punctuated an ongoing prayer session. Jodie, a somewhat lapsed Roman Catholic who was more likely to go to Methodist services with Steve than the church of her youth, had her late grandmother's rosary, and was clutching the worn beads, murmuring Hail Marys to herself. She remembered that her priest had required fifteen Hail Marys to atone for her transgressions when she was young, and she kept thinking, *If I say fifteen more, he'll be okay.* But then she lost count and started all over again. *Hail Mary, full of grace, the Lord is with you; blessed are you among women, and blessed is the fruit of your womb, Jesus. Holy Mary, Mother of God, pray for us sinners now and at the hour of our death. Amen.*

In the OR, Pegoli felt driven, knew that he had to get all of the tumor he could see, knew that right here was probably Grayson's only shot at growing up. In the cases that have been reported, survival rates are very low if any tumor is left behind and much more promising if no visible malignant cells remain. Even with his best effort, Pegoli knew that there might be tiny and virtually undetectable cancer cells left in Grayson, but they would be attacked with chemo and radiation later. Now he concentrated on excising every speck of the tumor he could find, knowing he had to work as efficiently as possible, with Grayson's blood pressure dropping and heart rate rising.

He reconstructed the portal vein with an allograft, a transplant from a tissue bank. That got blood flowing again, but the bowel was still so swollen that they couldn't close Grayson up. Grayson's organs, his stomach and part of the small intestine, were laid out on his abdomen, the organs and the opening covered with a transparent Gore-Tex patch. A respirator was breathing for him; he was barely stable. But Pegoli felt exhaustedly elated. It looked like his aggressive approach had paid off—he was pretty sure all the cancer was gone. The surgeon's exhilaration at having beat the cancer came through to Jodie and Steve as Pegoli explained the operation to them. He advised caution, but his excitement was contagious and Jodie and Steve dared to think positive thoughts again.

Still, it was hard to see Grayson in the recovery room and then the PICU (pediatric intensive care unit), on the respirator, the organs lying on his belly. *They're packing up these organs because he's going to die,* Jodie thought irrationally. He remained sedated, squirmed around a little, but his eyes didn't open. Steve counted eleven tubes in and out of his son's small body. *Is he going to make it, or isn't he?* Jodie rubbed his toes and fingers and talked softly in his ear, saying she loved him.

When she and Steve had to leave his bedside in the PICU, they left a tape playing softly—either recordings of them telling Grayson they loved him, or else his favorite song, "Bridge Over Troubled Water." It was appropriate. At the Christ statue the day after the operation, they were stunned to see that Grayson's note was still there and the one flower had multiplied—now there were dozens.

It seemed a hopeful portent but the next three days were studded with crises. First the superior mesenteric vein clotted, and Grayson was rushed back to the operating room so it could be cleared. Then three days after the big surgery, another clot appeared, this time in the portal vein. Again the doctors got blood flowing, and they were able to see that another healthy network of collateral blood vessels was growing to replace the vessels that had been consumed by tumor or obstructed with scar tissue. Finally the swelling subsided enough so that they were able to take off the patch, put Grayson's organs back in his abdominal cavity, hook his pancreas to his bowel, and close him up for good.

The days passed, and Jodie and Steve looked for sparks of life from Grayson. With the emergency surgeries in those first few days, it was a whole week before he was finally conscious enough to interact with anyone. His first words were to beg for a Coke. After fifteen days in the PICU he was moved back to a regular pediatric unit. Day by day, Steve and Jodie could see his strength returning. He didn't act very curious about what he had been through, and they told him simply that the lump in his tummy was gone. They didn't talk much about cancer. Grayson had seen enough to know that kids live and sometimes die with this disease. He was moving forward. He never asked, "Why me?" He passed his time watching movies and TV, coloring, drawing, snuggling with his parents, and getting better. He loved the regular trips in a wheelchair to the Jesus statue and felt that Jesus was watching over him.

Steve, too, got strength from the statue. He would look at it and get a feeling that it was made of more than marble. The figure touched the depths of his faith, the unshakable belief that there exists a spiritual energy that can provide strength. He sometimes talked quietly and unselfconsciously to The Divine Healer. He felt there was a force coming through, plain and clear. The beauty and simplicity gave him chills.

Dear Lord Jesus, please bless Grayson and may he live a long and healthy life. Our thoughts and prayers are with You. Love, Mom.
—APRIL, 1996

It was almost a smooth road as Grayson got back to living the life of a little boy again. Almost. After surgery, he had one more treatment with Adriamycin and cisplatin in April, and then got one dose of another potent chemo combination called VAC—vincristine, actino-mycin-D, and cyclophosphamide—the next month. No one wanted to take any chances, in case any errant cells had been left behind. Jodie and Grayson visualized the cancer cells as miniature Pac-Men, gobbling up all the healthy cells around them, and they wanted to get all of those greedy gluttonous Pac-Men out of there.

VAC is a powerful weapon that has demonstrated good results with a variety of cancers, but it packs a wallop of possible side effects, including damage to the liver, blood, and nerves. Steve was unavailable during most of the treatment period as Jodie watched Grayson go through a range of symptoms—complaints about leg soreness, muscle spasms in his fingers, fading vision, a cascade of worsening problems. It was the worst she'd ever seen him, except for immediately after the surgeries, and as the doctors asked her to step out of his hospital room while they treated him, she feared that after all this, he was going to die anyway. *Oh my God,* Jodie prayed out in the hallway, at the door to Grayson's room. *Please Lord, please save my baby. Please let him be healthy, we've gotten this far. I want to see him run, I want to see him grow.*

Grayson's electrolytes were seriously out of balance, the chemicals in the body that are essential for healthy human functioning. He was going into shock, and the doctors revived him with epinephrine, keeping close watch on his electrolyte levels so that they could provide the proper chemical balance through IV infusion. After hours of anxiety, Grayson stabilized enough for the chemo to resume, and did fine through the remainder of the treatment.

Jodie's relief was immense. When they left the hospital a few days later, the long and happy life that she prayed for at the statue actually seemed possible for Grayson. A photographer from the *Baltimore Sun* was there, and he took a picture of Grayson at the statue. For years to come, that photograph, which ran on the front page of the paper on Mother's Day, would remind Jodie of her son's vulnerability and innocence at that moment, but with the strength and power of the statue transfused to him.

The picture of Grayson at the statue was also a visible and permanent reminder to Jodie and Steve of the huge role that faith in God played in their son's recovery. They were amazed by the far-flung reports they heard of people praying for Grayson. They never doubted that their faith and the faith of hundreds of well-wishers, both known and unknown to them, had as significant a role in their son's recovery as the doctors' skills. In their minds, they equated the network of prayer that had been generated for Grayson with the network of collateral blood vessels that grew within his abdomen to keep his organs alive and healthy.

Other things were coming together. Somehow the Gilberts had managed to survive without income, supported by help from relatives and a financial outpouring from their community. A neighborhood women's co-op made meals, and neighbors contributed clothing and toys for the boys. A contribution box in Sherwood Market, a small grocery store a few blocks from their home, brought in $12,000 over the period of Grayson's treatment. The article in the *Sun* brought another round of contributions. The Grayson Gilbert fund was put together—even with healthcare coverage, the Gilberts ended up owing nearly $400,000. Because of the rarity of his disease, much of the treatment was considered experimental and not covered by their health plan.

After chemo, radiation seemed easy. It started in May and continued into July, five days a week, each session about an hour.

And then the treatment was over. There were a couple of happy respites, trips to western Maryland and Disney World donated by organizations that grant wishes of seriously ill children. At Disney World, the Give Kids the World foundation arranged for Grayson to meet his current favorite characters—Chip 'n' Dale had replaced Batman in Grayson's pantheon.

Today Grayson is recovered and healthy, but no battle of this magnitude ends without scars. "There are some pretty funky changes in there," a radiology resident remarked, seeing the interior of the boy's abdomen as the CAT scan images scrolled past on the computer monitor. Because much of his pancreas is gone, he takes digestive enzymes with his meals, and antacids and lactate to help further with digestion. An expensive multivitamin called ADEK needs to be special-ordered each month. So far, the remaining piece of pancreas has done a sufficient job of producing insulin, and Grayson's blood glucose remains in the normal range, but he is at risk for developing diabetes. He has a hearing loss from the cisplatin. He can hear normal speech, but misses high-frequency sounds like the sibilance of an *s*, the cymbals in a band, the complex high harmonics of a violin. His spleen is somewhat enlarged and has a tendency to consume blood cells, so his platelet count is low, but still within the normal range. Radiation may have caused sterility, but it will be years before that is known. At school, he sometimes has trouble concentrating, which may be related to the hearing loss.

Even these costs, though, are a small price to pay, because Grayson is alive. At ten, he is active, healthy, and growing, and as sweet-natured as he was five years ago. Jodie feels certain he has come through his ordeal because something special is meant for him in this world. His interests have turned to baseball, Babe Ruth to Cal Ripken, and he plays on a community league team. He is a talented artist and a number of his designs have been used on the Grant-A-Wish Foundation's Christmas cards. His sketchbook is full of drawings of Babe Ruth and Cal Ripken.

The Gilberts express their thanks and joy in prayers every day. And whenever they visit Hopkins, they pay a visit to The Divine Healer and leave a note for Him.

Dear Lord,

Thank You for Your love and healing towards our son Grayson Gilbert. It's been three years of happiness and bliss. Please, Lord, may he live to be a happy, healthy old man.

Love,
Mom & Dad
(Jodie and Stephen Gilbert)
Wes & Harrison too!
May 10, 1999

LEVI WATKINS, JR.
In His Hands

O Lord, my father's heart is in my hands, but his life, truly, is in Yours. Whatever the outcome here, I know it is Thy will. Lord, I pray Thy will be done.

In an operating room at The Johns Hopkins Hospital, cardiac surgeon Levi Watkins, Jr., held the heart of his father in his own hands and willed it to beat again. In his years of operating on hearts, his years of civil rights activism, his years of being a son and a brother and a physician, he had never before been so close to despair.

How did I get to this place? The question popped into his mind as he gently massaged the heart, something he had done many times before in his professional life. In the preceding minutes and hours, he had constructed three coronary artery grafts to bypass the blockage that prevented his father's blood from flowing adequately. He had repaired a faulty mitral valve. It seemed that every moment of his professional life—his training, his experience, his innovation, his years of perfecting techniques—had led him to this point. Even as he executed the technical details of surgery and directed the surgical team, he silently acknowledged God, his partner in the operation, and thanked Him for the skills that had put him in this place: *Dear God, there is nothing in the healing process greater than prayer.*

But then, as eighty-one-year-old Levi Watkins, Sr., was weaned from the heart-lung machine that kept his blood flowing and oxygenated during surgery, his heart failed to resume pumping on its own. Unable to generate the necessary blood pressure to push the blood out through the arteries into the body, the heart rapidly became engorged. "Quick, let's go back on the machine." Levi, Jr., snapped out the order, and as Jackie Martin, the anesthesiologist, pushed epinephrine into the IV line to jolt the heart into action, the surgeon cradled the organ in his hands and squeezed rhythmically in an attempt to stimulate beating again.

Had he done the wrong thing? There had been plenty of cautions against Levi, Jr., undertaking this procedure at all. Ethical guidelines in medicine clearly advise against a physician treating a family member. He knew some of his colleagues disagreed with what he was doing and were avoiding talking to him about his role in treating his father. Others had been more open in expressing their reservations.

His mother and sisters were concerned that if the surgery didn't work, he would forever blame himself. His own first reaction had been to say, "Daddy, you know I can't do this." But his brothers had strongly wanted him to do the procedure. And Daddy, himself, was adamant. He wanted none other than his son, internationally known cardiac surgeon Levi Watkins, Jr., M.D., to operate.

As his father's heart lay sluggish in his hand, images flitted through Levi, Jr.'s mind: his father taking him to the doctor to get a painful boil lanced when he was five; teaching him to drive on the family's 1960 Ford Galaxy, exhibiting his supreme patience as he waited until the last minute to grab the steering wheel to avert brushing a parked car; vigorously shaking his hand when Levi graduated medical school, not hugging him because that wasn't something Watkins men did. But Levi Watkins, Sr., inspired his three sons and three daughters with his integrity, his work ethic, his religiosity. Levi, Jr., was thrilled but humbled that his own gifts could be used to prolong his father's life. Had he now failed?

Dear Lord, Thy will be done with Daddy. Please, Lord, let me be the instrument of that will. He had prayed hard in the days before the surgery and felt as if he was calling on all the spirituality in him for support and affirmation. He had prayed for courage to do the right thing and for hope for his critically ill father. On the morning of the surgery, he had paused briefly at the foot of The Divine Healer, the statue he had come to know as a friend in his twenty-two years at Hopkins. He saw it as a tangible representation of that which was intangible, the faith in God that was an essential part of what he was as a man and as a surgeon. He didn't have much time—his team was waiting. *Just be with me if You will, Jesus,* he asked as he rubbed the glossy surface of the great toe.

And now in the OR, as the machine took over again, Levi, Jr., briefly felt something he had never felt before. He had considered worst-case scenarios and thought he had prepared himself mentally for the possibility of this moment. He was surprised at the fleeting sense of betrayal he felt. *God, how could You let this happen?* But that harsh, negative feeling was quickly replaced by the peace that prayer never failed to bring him. Whatever happened, it would be God's will.

If Levi Watkins, Jr., was one of the world's outstanding heart surgeons, it was because his father raised him to excel. Levi Watkins, Sr., the grandson of slaves, was born in 1911 in Montgomery, Kentucky, into a segregated world. Early in his life, he decided that the color of his skin would not be a barrier to achievement. From the time he could define his goals, he was determined that he would be a teacher, an educator who would imbue future generations, black and white, with the love of learning and the power of knowledge.

He got his bachelor's degree in 1933, majoring in mathematics at Tennessee A & I State College (now Tennessee State University), a school founded in 1912 to educate African Americans. He earned his master's degree in mathematics in 1940 at Northwestern University, in Illinois—leaving the predominately black higher education system and proving that he could easily hold his own scholastically with white folks. In 1940, he married Lillian Varnado, whom he met when they were both teaching at the same high school in Clarksville, Tennessee. They moved to Kansas where he taught junior high school mathematics and soon become principal of the school.

In 1948, Levi, Sr., moved his growing family to Montgomery, Alabama. He came back to Tennessee for a couple of years, from 1957 to 1959, and he founded S. A. Owen Junior College in Memphis. His last move was back to Montgomery, and in 1963 he became president of Alabama State University, where he would have his greatest professional impact. He led the school for nineteen years, until his retirement in 1981. A man who had fought and overcome obstacles all his life, he had a clear philosophy of how to succeed and prevail. He saw conflict and controversy as stepping stones to progress. He valued activism. "Nothing can be accomplished if all possible objections must first be overcome" read a plaque on his desk.

In his tenure at Alabama State, Levi, Sr., gained accreditation for the school, quadrupled the value of the physical plant, and sponsored a succession of students and faculty to earn advanced degrees. Many of these students stayed on or returned to teach at ASU. One of his greatest achievements was the upgrading of the faculty in his years of leadership. He set an example of indefatigable effort and sterling integrity. He was usually on the job every day. "We grew up thinking you were supposed to work seven days a week," remembers his fifth child, Donald, who became a lawyer. "I didn't know about a forty-hour work week until I went to work."

Levi, Sr., was also a devoted family man, although his time with his children was limited. It was Lillian who did the day-to-day child raising. There were two years between each of the six children—two girls, then Levi, Jr., then another sister and two brothers. Levi, Jr., remembers how his father assigned tasks to each of them—his were to take out the trash and shine everyone's shoes. On Sundays, the whole family would pile into the car and get ice cream. There wasn't a great deal of individual time for each child, but they all grew up knowing how important they were to their father and how much he cared for them. He was "Daddy" to all of them, even as adults. They grew up to become a mathematician, a teacher, a principal, a lawyer, and two surgeons, and each credited their father for much of their motivation to seek higher education and make a mark on the world.

Even as children, Levi and his brothers and sisters were aware of the segregation in their city and the discrimination faced by blacks. Montgomery was a city permeated with racial tension. Levi knew that he and other African Americans were not welcome at the movie theater, the municipal zoo, the swimming pool, the Dairy Queen. But Sundays at church, the First Baptist Church of Montgomery, his pastor Ralph David Abernathy preached a message of freedom and equal opportunity for black people. In 1955, the Watkins family switched to the Dexter Avenue Baptist Church and started hearing even more fiery sermons against segregation and intolerance by the young minister there. His name was Martin Luther King, Jr.

Later that year in Montgomery, the modern civil rights movement was sparked when Rosa Parks, a forty-two-year-old Montgomery seamstress, refused to give up her seat in the front of a bus to a white man. Her arrest precipitated a boycott of buses by blacks in the city. The boycott continued for nearly a year, until the U.S. Supreme Court declared that segregated seating on buses was unconstitutional. It was a volatile time. Blacks established carpools for themselves and were harassed by the police and snipers. A bomb was set off at Reverend King's home. King and other leaders of the boycott were charged with counts of conspiracy, and the minister was arrested on a petty speeding violation.

> But I trusted in Thee, O Lord,
> I said, Thou art my God.
> My times are in Thy hand,
> Deliver me from the hand of mine enemies,
> And from them that persecute me.

Hope

Make Thy face to shine upon Thy servant,
Save me for Thy mercies' sake.

—PSALMS 31:15–16

Young Levi was enthralled with the rhetoric and moved by the spirit of the battle for civil rights. He and other boys his age from the church formed a club called the Crusaders Club, which met evenings at Reverend King's house. With the eloquence that would soon become known to the nation, King spoke to the boys of the concept of God and the message of Christ, and how it connected to the civil rights movement. Levi knew this movement would remain a central force in his life. He was proud of his father's role as well, raising the caliber of his school and its students and taking direct action when necessary. He stood next to him as he faced down hooded, menacing Ku Klux Klansmen, when the school played in a stadium where blacks had never played before.

Levi, Jr., was valedictorian of his class at the Alabama State Laboratory High School. He was athletic, too, and was selected for the city of Montgomery's all-star basketball team. At Tennessee State University, his father's alma mater, he majored in biology and was president of the student body. Leadership came to him naturally and gracefully, part of his heritage from his dad. With his big Afro hairstyle and fervent opposition to intolerance, he had a reputation on campus as a firebrand but was also respected for his intelligence and civility. These were the years of the mid-sixties, the flowering of the civil rights movement, with conflicting emotional strains. There was the heady achievement of toppling barriers, an inexorable moving forward. But it was against a backdrop of pervasive and persistent ingrained prejudice and the ignorance and ugly hate that fueled it.

Young Levi thought he would follow in his parents' footsteps and become a teacher. In his senior year, his college adviser urged him to consider medicine—with his people skills and his aptitude for biology and the sciences, he was a natural, the professor said. Levi, Jr., liked the idea and started looking at medical schools. Both his parents were delighted that he wanted to be a doctor. Lillian wanted him to go to Meharry Medical College, in Nashville, a black school. It would be safe and noncontroversial and provide as good an education as any white school, she argued. But Levi, Jr., set his sights higher and his father agreed. They knew that to some white people, an M.D. from Meharry would not rate the same respect as a degree from an upper-echelon white school. He applied to Vanderbilt University School of Medicine, also in Nashville, and was accepted—the first black person to attend this respected institution.

Levi, Jr., wasn't particularly looking for the "first black" distinction, but he didn't avoid it either. With the intense demands of med school, working for social change took on a lesser priority, though the spirit of the movement was never far from Levi's heart. Well mannered and soft spoken, as Lillian had always insisted, he focused on his studies and ignored the few incidents of overt discrimination he encountered at Vanderbilt. But as the only black he was lonely, and he would never forget the terrible sense of isolation he felt on the tragic day in April 1968 when Martin Luther King, Jr., was assassinated. He could tell by their cavalier and thoughtless attitudes that none of his classmates shared his feelings or were even saddened by the assassination.

He was drawn to the discipline of surgery, and when he graduated from medical school in 1970, he decided to head north for internship and residency. Because of its reputation and the quality of its surgical training program, he chose Johns Hopkins. One of his first encounters at the hospital was with the Christ statue under the dome. The power of *Christus Consolator* stunned him the first time he saw it, and the impact of the presence didn't diminish through the years. It made him think of the healing powers of Jesus, of the many examples chronicled in the Bible. It also reminded him of the humanity of Jesus and the brotherhood of man, the principles to which he had devoted his efforts to achieve civil rights for black people. Finally, he thought of Jesus' activism. He was not presumptuous enough to compare his own actions to Christ's but he knew they were coming from a similar place. In his frequent contacts with the statue, these three strains were continually reinvigorated for him. Every time he saw The Divine Healer he was recommitted to what he was trying to do at Johns Hopkins and with his life in general. And he saw the statue as having a broad appeal and a message that transcended Christianity.

Levi, Jr., came to Maryland with high hopes of working in an integrated environment, where skin color would not be an issue. He should have known better. Yes, in Baltimore, he could go to the zoo and movie theaters, but housing and education were clearly segregated, not by law but by economics and social forces. The blacks he saw at Hopkins were much more likely to push brooms or serve food in the cafeteria than examine patients or guide scalpels. It was disappointing and troubling, and he knew that one day he would address the situation in some way. For the moment, though, he concentrated on becoming the best surgeon he could be. Increasingly, he was attracted by the challenges and opportunities offered by operating on the heart. Vincent Gott, then chief of cardiac surgery, mentored him and found him to be one of the finest surgeons he had ever supervised. In 1978, Levi became chief resident in cardiac surgery—the first black ever to hold the position, of course.

He took a break from surgery between 1973 and 1975 to study the mechanics of congestive heart failure in a physiology program at Harvard. His work helped define the chemical mechanism of the deadly disease, eventually leading to the use of angiotensin converting enzyme (ACE) inhibitors, medications that considerably improved the outlook for patients with congestive heart failure and other heart diseases.

Back at Hopkins, as his father was leading his own university into a new era, Levi, Jr., became a full-time faculty member in the division of cardiac surgery. And he assumed another role, recruiting qualified African-American students for the medical school. Richard

Ross, then dean of the medical school, designated Levi as a roving ambassador to travel the country and identify and interview the brightest minority students interested in studying medicine. In the years to follow, his efforts increased manyfold the number of black students who graduated from the Hopkins School of Medicine.

His surgical calendar was filled with bypasses, valve repairs, aneurysm repairs, and other procedures that are the crux of a cardiac surgeon's work. He became intrigued with the phenomenon of sudden death—unexplainable cardiac arrest. This usually occurs as a result of fibrillation, extremely rapid and uncoordinated contractions of some of the muscle fibers in the heart. When the heart stops in a medical setting, it can often be jolted back into action by applying electroshock through external defibrillator paddles. But 500,000 deaths a year in the United States were attributed to sudden cardiac arrest, primarily in people who arrest without medical resources close at hand. A Baltimore cardiologist, Michel Mirowski, had devised an implantable defibrillator that could be placed in people known to be at risk for sudden death. He had good results in the laboratory and was looking for a cardiac surgeon to start working with patients. Levi Watkins was interested, and the two began a collaboration that would save thousands of lives.

In February 1980, Levi implanted the first human automatic defibrillator, designed to detect very rapid, potentially lethal heart rhythms and immediately shock the heart back to a normal beat. In the following years, he continued to refine the procedure, and the device also evolved to increase utility and safety. Without a defibrillator, nearly one-third of all patients who survive one incident of sudden death end up dying within a year of another sudden cardiac arrest. Nearly all are dead within five years. But 95 percent of people with implantable defibrillators are alive and healthy five years after implantation.

Today the implantable defibrillator is a high-tech, streamlined version of the original model, and more than 100,000 lives have been saved by it. With the latest surgical innovations, the monitors that attach directly to the heart can be implanted through the subclavian vein in the shoulder without a chest incision, thus making the implantation procedure much less risky for the patient. Levi has personally implanted more than eight hundred defibrillators.

Levi, Jr., also had nonmedical accomplishments at Hopkins. In 1980, he established an annual Martin Luther King, Jr., commemoration that has brought international civil rights leaders to speak at Hopkins, including King's widow, Coretta Scott King, Nobel laureate Desmond Tutu, poet and author Maya Angelou, entertainers Harry Belafonte and Stevie Wonder, and his old friend Rosa Parks. (Parks had also become a patient, and Levi installed a pacemaker in her heart.) In the nineties, he began to divide his time between the operating room and the administrative offices of the medical school, serving as dean for postdoctoral programs, including internships and residencies.

As Levi, Jr.'s career was taking off, the elder Watkins's was winding down. He retired from the ASU presidency in 1981. But sometimes he was busier than he'd ever been, working as a consultant to ASU and other schools in the South. He also began writing a history of ASU. He and Lillian were growing old gracefully, enjoying their grandchildren and the success of their children. As they advanced through their seventies, they both were relatively healthy, although Levi, Sr., was treated for high blood pressure.

In summer 1992, Levi, Sr., became concerned about some swelling in his lower abdomen. Was he just gaining weight, or was something going on? His doctor had a CAT scan taken and diagnosed a benign cyst on the kidney. The doctor advised monitoring and a simple aspiration to relieve the pressure. "Feel this thing," Levi, Sr., said to his son when he was home for a late summer visit.

Levi, Jr., palpated his father's belly and didn't like the feel of it.

"That's pretty big," he said, and doubted it was just a cyst. "Why don't you come to Hopkins and we'll have someone there take care of this for you?"

In September, Levi, Sr., made the trip to Hopkins and was evaluated by urologist Fray Marshall. Marshall looked at a new set of CAT scans with radiologist Elliott Fishman, and they were fairly certain they were looking at a malignancy, not a cyst. They told Levi, Jr., and it was he who told his parents that it looked like Daddy had cancer. Levi, Sr., and Lillian were shocked—they had thought this was something minor. In the living room of Levi, Jr.'s townhouse on the Baltimore waterfront, the three of them prayed together. Lillian's favorite psalm was the twenty-third, and they repeated the familiar words again and again:

> *O Lord,*
> *Yea, though I walk through the valley of the shadow of death*
> *I will fear no evil*
> *For Thou art with me.*
> *Thy rod and Thy staff they comfort me.*
>
> —PSALMS 23:4

His father was not the first patient Levi, Jr., prayed for and with. Through the years, many of his patients learned of the heart surgeon's deep faith in God, and some had asked him to pray with them. He'd taken some to see the Christ statue, or prayed with them in the small chapel off the Children's Center lobby. Prayer was something the surgeon wrapped around himself like a cloak—he felt very lonely and exposed without it. His parents felt the same way.

Marshall scheduled a radical nephrectomy (complete removal of the kidney) for Levi, Sr., on September 14, 1992. Levi, Jr., waited with his mother and five brothers and sisters, who had come together at their father's bedside. It was hard waiting—*I'd rather be the one doing the surgery than waiting,* Levi, Jr., thought prophetically. A couple of hours into the procedure, he talked to Marshall, a friend as well as colleague, and the urologist told him he wasn't sure he could get all the cancer out. But the pathology lab found clean margins around the tumor—it looked like the cancer had been contained and all removed.

Levi, Jr.'s five brothers and sisters were all in the Hopkins waiting room with their mother, and they heard the news together. Their prayers this time were of joyful thanks.

Praise ye the Lord.
We give thanks unto the Lord
for He is good
and His mercy endureth
forever.

—PSALMS 106:1

The elderly often recuperate slowly, and Levi, Sr., was no exception, but during the first six days after the surgery he made steady progress. One night a week after the operation, Levi, Jr., was home in bed when he got a middle-of-the-night call from the hospital. At first he thought the resident was telling him one of *his* patients had experienced a cardiac arrest. Then he realized the doctor was talking about his father.

He was at the hospital within minutes, not wanting to intimidate the team working on his father, but needing to be on the scene. "You're doing good, you're doing real good," he murmured to the resident. Levi, Sr., was stabilized and moved first to the surgical intensive care unit, then the coronary care unit. An echocardiograph found a clot and poor function of the left ventricle, the chamber of the heart that pumps the blood to the body. Levi, Sr., had suffered a serious heart attack. Recovery was a "complicated course," cardiologist Steven Schulman, director of the CCU, wrote later to Levi, Sr.'s Montgomery doctor. He developed an infection, and then bleeding in his stomach and small intestine. But medications solved these problems, the chest pain and shortness of breath went away, and within another two weeks Levi, Sr., was walking the halls and ready to go home.

He took it easy at home, appreciating the severity of his condition. He was taking nine different medications daily, but started to get around more and think about getting back to work on the college history. But on November 2, less than a month after he'd been discharged from Hopkins, he was admitted to a local hospital with shortness of breath and irregular heartbeat. Another heart attack. When he talked to his father's doctor on the phone, Levi, Jr., knew he had to get his father back to Hopkins so he could see exactly what was going on and help his parents make decisions about the best course of treatment.

Levi, Sr., was readmitted to Hopkins and on November 25 underwent cardiac catheterization, a diagnostic procedure in which a tube (catheter) is inserted through a blood vessel in the groin and threaded up to the heart. Then a dye visible in X-rays is injected into the catheter, allowing a clear view of blood flow patterns. Levi, Sr.'s catheterization showed severe blockage of three coronary arteries, and malfunction of the mitral valve. He needed surgery. And he knew who he wanted to do it—his son.

Treatment of immediate family members has long been considered a questionable practice for physicians. In November 1992, when Levi, Jr., and his family were making the decision that he would operate on his father's heart, the American Medical Association had no specific stated policy on the issue. Historically, the AMA had explicitly advised against physicians treating their own family members. But in 1977, the AMA Judicial Council (now the Council on Ethical and Judicial Affairs) revised its guidelines and omitted any mention of treatment of family members as "historical anachronism." In June

1993, the Council did address the issue with a policy statement that concluded, "Physicians generally should not treat themselves or members of their immediate families."

In 1992, eight months before Levi, Jr., decided to operate on his father, the *Journal of the American Medical Association* published an article suggesting that physicians consider seven questions when making a decision about treating family members: (1) Am I trained to meet my relative's medical needs? (2) Am I too close to probe my relative's intimate history and to cope with bearing bad news? (3) Can I be objective enough to give appropriate care? (4) Is medical involvement likely to provoke or intensify conflicts within the family? (5) Will relatives comply with medical directives from a family member? (6) Will I allow referral for treatment to another physician? (7) Am I willing to be accountable to my peers and the public for this care?

Levi, Jr.'s immediate reaction to his father's request that he do the surgery was negative—based on the ingrained notion that it just wasn't done. In fact, it is frequently done—the 1992 *JAMA* article published data showing that doctors often examine, diagnose, and prescribe medications for family members. This survey found that 11 percent of the doctors questioned had operated on family members. And there was historic precedent within his own institution: William Halsted, Hopkins's famed first chief of surgery, had removed his mother's gallbladder.

When Levi, Jr., considered the seven questions, he didn't have trouble with any of them. Clearly, he was trained to meet his father's medical needs—he was one of the top heart surgeons at one of the best hospitals in the world. Intimacy was not an issue, nor was objectivity or family conflict or compliance. As the surgeon, he worked on a team with cardiologists and intensivists, who would be involved in the postsurgical care. And he was certainly willing to be accountable for his actions.

His mother and sisters were concerned that if Levi, Sr., died on the operating table, Levi, Jr., would blame himself. Levi, Jr., thought it through and concluded that his training and experience and spirituality had prepared him to face this burden. The more he thought about it, and prayed about it, the more he felt that it was no accident that his life's work had brought him to this decision. He felt this was something God meant him to do. At eighty-one, with his medical problems, Levi, Sr., wouldn't have a second chance to have his heart fixed. This was his only opportunity. Everyone who loved him wanted to make sure he got the best possible treatment.

Levi, Jr., didn't consult many of his colleagues about what he was planning, but he did talk to Vince Gott, the senior heart surgeon at Hopkins and his mentor. Gott was a little surprised but supportive. He knew that if there was any heart surgeon who could handle the emotional stress of operating on a family member, it was Levi Watkins, Jr. Gott agreed to assist in the surgery.

Once the decision was made, Levi, Jr., knew he had to prepare himself emotionally and spiritually. He didn't underestimate the task. He found himself praying as he walked the halls of the hospital and spending more time than usual at church. He discussed the matter at length with his pastor, Vernon Dobson, and they prayed together. His prayers were general and free floating—Levi had learned through the years not to pray for specific things. *Please, God, Thy will be done with Daddy. God, let me carry out that will. And God, please give me the strength to deal with whatever comes, whether it is good or bad.*

The surgery was scheduled for November 30. As the day approached, Levi, Jr., distanced himself from his father. He was surgeon first, son second. For a couple of days before the operation, he did not see his father at all, although he did remain apprised of his medical status. He was not with Lillian and his brothers and sisters—again gathered at their father's bedside—as they kissed the old man, squeezed his hand, and watched him be wheeled down the corridor to the operating room. In the scrub area, Levi, Jr., waited until the last possible moment, until his father was fully prepped and draped and his chest open, to enter the operating room. He approached his father's heart exactly as he had approached the thousands of hearts he had held in his hands in his years of operating. He had healed many a damaged heart and he silently asked God to help him heal another.

The surgery went routinely and his father remained stable—until it was time for his heart to start beating on its own again. Then the heart was filling but not emptying. *It's blowing up,* Levi, Jr., thought, and for a moment almost panicked. In those few alarming minutes as he thought God had let him down, he squeezed the heart and said to himself, *This could be our worst-case scenario happening right here.* He envisioned telling his family that Daddy had died on the operating table, the pain they all would feel. He thought of what some of his colleagues might say, or think.

But neither of these were his concerns now—now, he needed to remain totally focused on getting the heart to beat. As he ordered the bypass machine started again and consulted with the anesthesiologist about the doses of heart-stimulating drugs, he felt the despair leave him, replaced by a calm certainty that God's will would be done and that was all he could hope for.

Later he thought simply and thankfully, *The will was there.* As the epinephrine raced through Levi Sr.'s bloodstream, the heart picked up the rhythm of Levi, Jr.'s squeezing hands and gained strength. Once again the patient was weaned from the heart-lung machine, and this time his heart was up to the challenge. Levi, Jr., wanted to jump for joy. *Better stay cool, better stay professional,* he reminded himself, and he kept his emotion contained as his father's chest was closed and he was taken to the recovery room.

Unto Thee, O Lord, do we give thanks;
Unto Thee do we give thanks

In His Hands

For that Thy name is near
Thy wondrous works declare.

—PSALMS 75:1

Levi, Sr.'s recovery was slow, to be expected in an elderly person undergoing such a serious procedure. But there was steady improvement and a gradual reduction in doses of the medications that supported his heart. He was discharged on Christmas Day 1992, and Levi, Jr.—along with two of his sisters and three of their children—accompanied his parents on the plane to Montgomery. His father was frail, but gaining strength every day and filled with joyful prayerfulness at being alive.

On December 26, the Watkins offspring surprised their parents with an oft-delayed fiftieth anniversary party. Both Lillian and Levi, Sr., spoke emotionally to the family and friends who had gathered. Sitting next to each other on the couch under a sign that said "Congratulations for 50 years of exciting love," they thanked God and their son that he had lived to see this day. "My kids know from whence their help comes," Lillian began. ". . . The Man upstairs knew I needed lots of help and didn't mind asking. I learned from my father as a very young one about prayer. We had it every morning around the breakfast table. So whether we knew we were absorbing it or not, we were, and it just stuck and stuck and stuck."

As Lillian gently rubbed his head and neck, Levi, Sr., spoke with an emotion that his children had rarely seen. "The psalmist once asked, 'What is man that Thou art mindful of him?' At Johns Hopkins Hospital, when I realized after surgery that I was alive, and that I had a chance perhaps to live, I asked the question, why me? Why did God save me? I came to know through that crisis the strength of my family in ways perhaps I would never have known and in ways perhaps few men will ever know. I saw them pray.

". . . In that critical moment and for that critical need, God has given me—why me?—a son who had the skill, the ability to do what needed to be done and the courage to do it."

And then Levi (Alec) Garroway, their oldest grandson, played Levi, Sr.'s favorite prayer on the violin. One by one, family members joined in and sang the Lord's Prayer:

Our Father
Who art in heaven,
Hallowed be Thy name.
Thy kingdom come,
Thy will be done
On earth as it is in heaven.

In the following months, Levi, Sr., got back to work on the history of ASU he was writing. His heart was weakening, though, and he had only one kidney—he knew his remaining days were limited. Through 1993, medical tests showed his heart gradually enlarging and he was beginning to develop shortness of breath, swelling of his ankles, and irregular heartbeat—symptoms of congestive heart failure. In a visit with his Montgomery doctor in June 1993, Lillian told him that her husband was "working relentlessly" to finish his book. Later that year, when Levi, Jr., was home on a visit, father and son had an unemotional talk about how the old man wanted to die. "Don't ever let me *not* be Levi Watkins," he told his son, and Levi, Jr., agreed.

Levi, Sr., was admitted to a Montgomery hospital in late February 1994 with congestive heart failure and kidney failure. The months since his son had operated on his heart had been productive and joyful ones—he'd celebrated his fiftieth wedding anniversary, finished his book, worked as a consultant, seen a new great-grandchild, bought a new car. He died on March 3, age 83. The death was quiet and peaceful, and he passed away surrounded by his wife and children. When she realized he had taken his last breath, Lillian lay across his body and wept. Levi, Jr., was dry-eyed, grateful that Daddy had the peace he deserved.

On the morning of the funeral, four days later, the galleys of the book were delivered to the house. No one in the family had seen them, no one knew that the book was dedicated to Levi, Jr., a father's last act of gratitude to a son for extending his life. "[W]ith God's will and the skill of my son, Levi, Jr., . . . I have survived," he wrote in the Prologue. "With their help I have been given an extended lease on life and strength for the rigors of further research."

Levi, Jr., was surprised, humbled, and proud, and with his family prayed for his father's eternal peace:

> *The Lord is my light and my salvation;*
> *Whom shall I fear?*
> *The Lord is the strength of my life;*
> *Of whom shall I be afraid?*
> *Wait on the Lord,*
> *Be of good courage,*
> *And He shall strengthen thine heart.*
> *Wait, I say, on the Lord.*

—PSALMS 27:1, 14

*M*iracle Michaila

God gives us
so many wonderful things,
the promise of healing,
the comfort of prayer,
and the dearest of blessings,
His own loving care

——GREETING CARD, FRAMED AND HUNG
IN PAUL AND KATE DISNEY'S LIVING ROOM

Michaila Disney was born with eyes that did not see and ears that did not hear. Her intestinal tract had no exit from her body and her heart had three holes in it. Her brain was so crowded in her head by excess cerebrospinal fluid that it looked like only a small fraction of a normal-size brain.

The human body is an amazing interacting combination of systems, each fulfilling its specialized task. The miracle of all these systems working together properly is normal, commonplace human life. In Michaila Disney, nearly none of the systems worked as they are supposed to. But Michaila has lived and developed and grown. By age three, she had progressed beyond what many experts predicted would be possible for her. At The Johns Hopkins Hospital, where she has benefited from state-of-the-art technology and care from more than a half-dozen pediatric specialties, she is called Miracle Michaila.

~

"Silly, silly baby." Kate Disney, Michaila's mother, tickles her daughter under the chin and laughs along with Michaila's little giggle.

Seated in her high chair, Michaila rummages around the cookie pieces and cheese crackers on her tray with her hands and brings a piece to her mouth. She chews and swallows, then grabs her bib with her hands and tugs at it. "Okay, now, little Miss Bird," Kate croons to her. Dressed in a yellow jumpsuit, her unruly brown hair pulled into a scrunchy at the top of her head, Michaila covers her rosy cheeks with her hands and starts to rock rhythmically in her chair.

"She's tired," Kate says, reaching for Michaila, who wraps her arms around her mother's neck. "Nap time, little one." Kate hands Michaila to Paul, and the little girl settles into a comfortable snuggle on her father's shoulder. It is a familiar position for her—Paul, who works for a software company, spends many hours at the home computer and often holds Michaila on his shoulder as he works.

They live in a small powder-blue ranch house half a mile down an unpaved driveway in a community south of Annapolis, Maryland. Paul steps quietly as he lays Michaila in her youth bed; he doesn't want to wake her roommate, eight-month-old Rachel. Michaila, at three, is the oldest of three siblings—in the middle is two-year-old Nathaniel, a walky-talky bundle of energy who runs circles around his sisters, one because of her age, the other because of her disabilities.

Nathaniel and Rachel were unplanned children—Paul and Kate, barely out of their teens when Michaila was born, knew they would be busy enough with their first. But even though the pregnancies were unplanned, the babies could not have been more wanted. Maybe this unexpected fertility was God's plan, Paul and Kate have come to believe. Because nothing could be more valuable to helping Michaila develop than to have two close-in-age siblings progressing normally through their developmental milestones.

Life with one child with multiple handicaps and all three in diapers can be stressful. You couldn't find two people better equipped to handle it than Paul and Kate Disney. Kate is super-organized, with a diaper bag always packed for each kid, lists for the tasks she has to accomplish each day. Paul is organized in his own way; his reaction to life events and crises—engagement, marriage, Michaila's birth, the other children following so quickly behind—has been to work out a budget, anticipate the family's needs, and figure out how he will meet them.

But faith and prayer are the main tools they rely on to cope. Looking over Paul's shoulder as he lays Michaila in her bed, Kate speaks softly of the role it plays. "Without prayer, we never could have handled everything we've gone through with Michaila," she says. "Everything in our life has followed prayer. Prayer has confirmed things for us when we needed confirmation. God has never been too late, never been too early. He always shows up right in the nick of time, through other people or some sort of sign. He has never let us down."

Paul Disney and Katherine Packett both grew up within a few miles of their current home. They met in August 1991, when he was sixteen and she seventeen, at Sunday service at Edgewater Baptist Church. Kate's father, who made a midlife career switch from the insurance industry to the ministry, had just finished the seminary and assumed duties as an associate pastor at the church. He asked his family to be with him at his first Sunday service. Kate didn't want to go. She had recently returned from a missionary trip to Appalachia and wanted to speak about her mission that Sunday at the Church of God she had grown up in. But she would not refuse her father's request.

Paul, who came to church every Sunday with his family, was with his brother and some friends in a back pew. When Kate walked in with her parents, Paul stared at this bouncy-haired, self-assured girl. She sat in the front row with her mother, sister, and brothers, and he managed to be introduced after the service. Despite his clean-cut good looks, she didn't take much notice of him until they started running into each other at the weekly meetings of the church youth group. Kate was cautious about dating him—he was a year younger, which seemed important at this age. But in the youth group she was attracted to his spirit for the Lord, so similar to her own. In October, she asked him to go with her to a party at her school, the Annapolis Area Christian School. From then on they were together on weekends and whenever they could manage during the week.

After high school, Paul and Kate attended Anne Arundel Community College. They were in love and wanted to get married. At eighteen and nineteen, they knew they were young, but they felt sure of their path. Together and apart, they prayed for guidance to do the right thing. *Lord, show us Your will, give us wisdom to make the right choices.* Paul was in school full time and worked part time, selling shoes on commission. Kate worked full time and was in school part time. They decided if they could find a place with rent less than four hundred dollars a month and Kate could get a job making seven dollars an hour, they could afford to get married. They prayed on it. *Lord, show us a place to live if this is Your will. You know our resources, show us a place where we can live together on our modest means.*

Within weeks Kate got a better-paying job as office manager for a landscaping business and they saw an ad for the little rancher for four hundred dollars. They felt the pieces of their lives were falling into place. They sat down with both sets of parents, showed them their budget and their plans, asked their approval and received it. They got engaged on April 1, 1994, and married August 13 the same year.

The house was a mess, with holes in the floor, tiny nonfunctional windows, ugly metal siding, and soiled worn carpet. But the landlord agreed to pay for supplies if Paul and Kate did the necessary improvement work themselves. They gutted the place and fixed it up, from outdoor siding to new windows to inside paneling and flooring. It was exhausting work and consumed their spare time, but they were having fun. They thanked God for their good fortune in finding each other and for the sanctity of their love.

Kate wanted to get pregnant almost right away, but Paul, more cautious, thought they should wait. After a year and a half, they decided it was time. Kate found out she was pregnant while shopping with her mother in the Annapolis Mall. She took a home pregnancy test in the mall bathroom, and when she told her mom it was positive, they switched from shopping for a chair to looking for baby things. Kate bought Paul a bib that said, "I love my daddy," and gave it to him with the pregnancy test result. He hugged her with joy. "I've got to make a new budget," he told her.

No testing has overtaken you that is not common to man. God is faithful and He will not suffer you to be tested beyond your strength; but with the testing, He will also provide the way out so that you may be able to endure it.

—I CORINTHIANS 10:13

Kate had morning sickness all day long and it continued beyond the usual first trimester. But that didn't diminish her happiness about having a baby, and Paul was excited too, in his more reserved way. When she was eighteen weeks pregnant, he took off work to accompany her for her first sonogram. With a wand, the radiology technician pointed out the body parts on the monitor. "These are the feet, these are the hands." Then she stopped talking for a moment. *This silence does not feel good*, Kate thought, and a sense of dread began to grow. Later she thought of it as mother's intuition.

"What's the matter?" she asked.

"Nothing," answered the technician, turning the screen away. "I'm going to get the doctor."

Kate was not usually a crier, but tears ran down her cheeks as the technician left the room and she and Paul looked at each other in alarm. The doctor came in, examined the image with the technician, and turned to Paul and Kate. "It's probably nothing to worry about," she said. "It looks like there's a pocket of fluid in the brain, but it's likely it will reabsorb before the baby is born." She said she would consult with a radiologist and talk to them more in a day or two.

The reassurance sounded false to Kate and Paul, and they left the doctor's office feeling confused and fighting panic. When Paul called the doctor back, she admitted she was concerned, but she wasn't prepared to talk about it until she consulted the radiologist. The next day she called Kate at work.

It was Thursday, June 20, 1996, the day the Olympic torch relay passed through Maryland on its way to open the summer Olympics in Atlanta. Kate's firm was located on Route 2, the route of the relay, and her office overlooked the highway. As she talked to the doctor on the phone, her office filled with people looking out the window, and she clapped a hand over her ear to block the sound of her coworkers cheering. She would never forget the irony of hearing cheers in one ear and news worse than anything she expected in the other.

The obstetrician told Kate that her fetus was hydrocephalic, it looked like a serious case, and the baby probably wouldn't live. "You're young," the doctor said, and Kate knew she was trying to be compassionate but the words offered no solace. "You should reconsider things right now. There are ways to terminate the pregnancy, and you won't have to deal with this anymore."

For Thou has possessed my reins; Thou hast covered me in my mother's womb.
I will praise Thee; for I am fearfully and wonderfully made: marvelous are Thy works; and that my soul knoweth right well.
My substance was not hid from Thee when I was made in secret, and curiously wrought in the lowest parts of the earth.
Thine eyes did see my substance, yet being unperfect; and in Thy book all my members were written, which in continuance were fashioned, when as yet there was none of them.

—PSALMS 139:13–16

Kate and Paul prayed that night, but neither felt the need to ask for guidance about abortion. It was not an option. They decided to switch to a doctor who shared their feelings, and through their church network found Clifton McClain, an obstetrician in nearby Pasadena. They learned that hydrocephalus, an excess of cerebrospinal fluid in the brain, is not uncommon, and treatments allow many children with this condition to live normal lives. As the pregnancy advanced, Kate had weekly sonograms. Every week she would pray for the same thing: *Lord, could You please let this baby live? Please, Lord, let them look now and see it is improved. Let all that fluid be gone this time when the doctor looks. If it's gone, I'll tell the whole world what You have done for me.*

But sonograms showed the hydrocephalus progressively worsening. McClain referred Kate and Paul to a pediatric neurosurgeon at Children's Hospital in Washington, D.C., so they could learn more about the implications of fetal hydrocephalus. They saw him when Kate was twenty-two weeks pregnant. He said the same thing they had heard from the first obstetrician: "You're young, you can try again. Abortion is your best course." *We're looking for solutions, and he's telling us to bail out,* Kate thought bitterly. If they decided not to abort, the doctor added, they should start looking for institutions where they could place the baby.

Kate and Paul were frightened but not disheartened. They refused to believe there was no chance their baby would be normal. Paul couldn't understand how cavalier the doctors were about this tiny life. All the consideration went to him and Kate, they were young, they shouldn't have to deal with this, and on and on. *What about the baby?* he asked himself. *Why was no consideration given to the baby?*

Lots of bad things happen in life, he thought, *but they don't always have bad results. God uses weak things as a reflection of His own strength. He uses weak things to put to shame the strong. If we were to play God, to end this life, then a blessing would be missed, a purpose wouldn't be served. I don't have the right to do that.*

They wanted to find another neurosurgeon to talk to about what they could do. Kate's aunt had recently interviewed pediatric neurosurgeon Benjamin Carson for the newsletter of the Bethany Christian Services, a national organization that offers pregnancy counseling and adoption services. She told Kate and Paul about him. Carson was nearby, just forty miles north at The Johns Hopkins Hospital in Baltimore. And he was known not only for his outstanding surgical achievements, but also for his Christian faith and inspirational work. Kate called his office and made an appointment.

From their first meeting, Carson gave Kate and Paul the hope they were looking for. "This is the Lord's child," he said, echoing their own feelings. He made them feel he respected them and their beliefs. "Medicine, for the most part, makes logical sense," he told them. "If someone tells you something that doesn't make sense, you should question it."

Carson gave them a pamphlet to read about the ventriculo-peritoneal shunt, the most common treatment for hydrocephalus. The VP shunt is a thin, surgically implanted tube that drains CS fluid from the ventricles of the brain, the cavities where the fluid builds, to the peritoneal area in the abdomen, where it is absorbed naturally. Many hydrocephalic children have normal intelligence and development, Paul and Kate read in the pamphlet. But it also said that sometimes hydrocephalus causes mental retardation.

"Paul," Kate said, "do you think the baby will be retarded?"

"I don't know," he answered, and they prayed together. *God,* Kate thought, *I think we can handle just about everything, but there are three things I don't know if we can handle. I don't know if we can handle a wheelchair, or mental retardation, or bowel problems.* She didn't know why those three types of disabilities came to mind, but at the time they seemed like overwhelming burdens to her.

Another night they watched a TV movie about two young blind people who met each other and married. Kate started crying. "What if the baby's blind?" she sobbed. "Why are you worrying about that?" Paul chided her. "If she's blind, the Lord will get us through that too."

⁓

Do not be anxious about anything, but in everything, by prayer and petition, with thanksgiving, present your requests to God. And the peace of God, which transcends all understanding, will guard your hearts and your minds in Christ Jesus.
—PHILIPPIANS 4:6–7

The sonograms showed that the ventricles in the baby's brain were getting bigger. Carson had told them that the baby would soon be viable, and labor would be induced as soon as he and David Nagey, the perinatologist (high risk pregnancy specialist), thought it was safe for her to be born. It would not be long.

When Kate was in her seventh month, "Pat" Packett—her father and pastor—brought her and Paul to the front of the congregation he now led, the Chesapeake Christian Fellowship. This nondenominational church didn't have its own building but met for services at a local high school. Kate's father had arranged a prayer for healing during the service. He gave the worshipers a brief explanation of his daughter's situation—most of them knew already. Then he asked the elders of the church to come forward, and they touched Kate and Paul and prayed. They prayed for the healing of the baby, they prayed that Kate would be able to endure the birth, they prayed that Paul and Kate would be able to handle whatever the Lord had in store.

Then Paul spoke. "We are all putting our hearts into praying for healing," he said, "but we have to remember, this might not be healing that we can understand. Just because it doesn't turn out the way we think it should doesn't mean we should stop praying. We all need to keep our faith, whatever the outcome."

Hope

The healing service filled Kate with a tremendous peace, the peace she had read about in Philippians, a peace that surpasses all understanding. *It will all be okay,* she thought. *Whatever God gives us, it will be okay.*

After a sonogram toward the end of September, Nagey called and said the baby's head was getting dangerously large—it was time for her to be born. Kate was thirty-four weeks pregnant, more than a month short of full term, but it had become more dangerous for the baby to remain in utero than to be born prematurely. Kate, with Paul and all four of their parents, were at Hopkins at five P.M., September 30, to "ripen" her cervix. The cervix is the thick conical plug at the bottom of the uterus that keeps a fetus in place during pregnancy. In order for the baby to move into the birth canal, the cervix must efface (thin out) and dilate (open up), becoming softer and more pliable. Kate's cervix was neither effaced nor dilated, so a combination of mechanical and hormonal treatment was tried. It was very painful for Kate. By midnight she was effaced but still hadn't begun to dilate. The doctor told her to go home, get a few hours sleep, come back at six A.M. the next day, and labor would be induced.

Kate and Paul prayed more than they slept that night and arrived at the hospital on October 1. Paul carried an overnight bag for Kate and another packed with clothes for the baby to wear home. Labor was induced with intravenous Pitocin, and the contractions began, quick and intense from the start. But there was little progress, and the drug was stopped in the evening to give the contracting uterus a rest. Kate spent that night in the hospital and in the morning the Pit drip, as it is called, began again. During an internal sonogram, which showed the baby holding her hands over her eyes, Kate's water broke. She was pushing but the labor was not progressing, and the doctors decided to perform a cesarean section.

Nearly a dozen obstetricians, anesthesiologists, neonatologists, nurses, and technicians filled the delivery room. The epidural (local) anesthetic Kate had been given wasn't taking hold as it should and she was given general anesthesia. Paul held her hand; she was very frightened. "Please don't let me and my baby die," she begged the anesthesiologist and then turned to her husband. "Paul, pray for me and the baby."

Michaila was born at 10:34 P.M., October 2, 1996, weighing four pounds, five ounces. Paul watched the doctor remove her and was surprised at how blue she was. As he looked and listened, she let out a cry, which tapered into breathlessness. He was concerned but calm as he watched. The baby was taken to a warming table and he saw her skin take on a pinker tone as the doctors worked on her.

But here was a surprise—the sonograms had indicated that the baby was a girl but at birth one of the doctors announced, "It's a boy." *I wonder how they got it wrong on so many sonograms,* Paul reflected, but that seemed a minor issue. What was important was that the baby was alive, and now he needed to know more about its condition—he could see some red marks on the face and thought it was blood. The Isolette wheeled past, taking the baby to the neonatal intensive care unit. There weren't any tubes hooked up yet, and that seemed to be a good sign. He had a fleeting impression that one eye looked bigger than the other, but thought, *I don't have much experience with this, I don't know what newborns are supposed to look like. Maybe this is normal.*

About forty-five minutes after the birth, Paul was in the recovery room with Kate when the doctors said they were ready to talk to him about his baby's condition. Leaving Kate with her mother, he went to the NICU where Frances Northington, the attending neonatologist, and two residents gently but bluntly ticked off for Paul a list of all the things wrong with his baby. First of all, they said, the baby had eye problems and would probably be blind. It also had an "imperforate anus," which means absence of a normal opening. He already knew about the hydrocephalus. The red skin was caused by something called dermal aplasia, defective development of the skin and blood vessels. These problems were probably part of a syndrome, a collection of abnormalities, the doctors went on, and hearing impairment was likely to be another of the disabilities. Finally, the baby had ambiguous genitalia—it was impossible to tell by looking whether it was a boy or girl.

Paul felt overwhelmed, stunned. He seized on what he hadn't heard. "How are the heart and lungs?" he asked. "Is the heart beating, is he stable? Can I see him?"

See *him?* After thinking about the baby as a girl for five months, it was hard to make this sudden switch. Was it a boy or a girl? They couldn't even give it a name. What would they tell other people? It seemed an especially cruel problem. It would take two weeks before results of a chromosome test would provide definitive information. In the nursery it just said Baby Disney over the Isolette.

Since they had said it was a boy when it was born, Paul decided to think of it as *him*. He visited for about a half hour after the doctors told him all the bad news. He held the baby's hand, rubbed its arm, wondered how the baby was perceiving him. The infant didn't look as bad as all those problems the doctors had listed. The name they had chosen for a boy was Nathaniel. "I'm your daddy, how are you doing, Nathaniel?" Paul whispered. The baby was hooked up to a ventilator, and there were intravenous lines and monitors attached to the little body. "I'm so glad you're here, we've been praying for you," Paul continued. "You are going to be fine, and your mommy and daddy love you very much." One of the nurses had a Polaroid camera, and he took a picture to show Kate.

It was too soon, Paul decided, to have the painful discussion with Kate about the uncertainty of the baby's gender. He told her the baby had eye problems and was on a ventilator and stable. He showed her the photo; Kate was alarmed at the red skin. She, too, felt overwhelmed. She threw up throughout the day following the birth and felt miserable. Paul made several trips in the next two days to the NICU to spend time with the baby, but Kate was afraid to go.

By evening of the baby's second day, it was extubated, breathing on its own, and gaining a little weight. Dr. Nagey told Paul and Kate that he feared the baby had a condition called holoprosencephaly, characterized by failure of the brain to properly divide into two hemispheres. Brain development in these children is often severely impaired, and they usually don't live past infancy. The diagnosis was based on an MRI of the baby's brain, which remained compressed by the excess cerebrospinal fluid. Kate couldn't take it in; when the doctor left, she turned from Paul and drifted into sleep, still dopey from the painkillers she was taking. Paul, who had spent time with the baby, could think of the person, not just the diagnosis. When he saw Kate awakening, he leaned over and whispered, "Will you please come down and see the baby with me? If you look at the child, you can deal with the diagnosis, no matter what they tell us."

Kate wasn't sure she could love something she couldn't understand. How could she relate to this baby who couldn't see or hear her? But she let Paul help her out of bed and into a wheelchair, and he pushed her down the corridor to the NICU. As soon as she saw her baby, her fears about loving it and relating to it evaporated. *It's just a baby,* she thought, *a cute little baby.* The redness on the face had faded. She looked down on a very lovable newborn. How could she have doubted it?

In the NICU, Paul and Kate held hands and prayed:

We give thanks, Lord, for this baby's life. Please Lord, heal his blindness, allow him to poop, fix his skin. Allow our baby to remain whole, allow the brain to remain stable so that at the right time Dr. Carson can fix it. Give us strength, give us wisdom, to deal with all the problems this child will have. Thank You, Lord.

When Kate thought about it later, she laughed at her naivete in packing clothes for her newborn to wear home. This baby would be in the hospital for weeks, maybe even months. It faced numerous surgeries on several of its tiny systems. An exit was needed for Michaila's digestive system, but that formed spontaneously shortly after birth, and no medical intervention was necessary. Called a peritoneal fistula, it didn't have much muscle control, but it would serve the purpose for at least two years when more surgery would put in a more permanent exit.

When the baby was only a couple days old, involvement of yet another system was found—an echocardiogram turned up three holes in the heart. These defects seemed like a dizzying array of initials to Kate and Paul—PDA, VSD, ASD. The letters are short for patent ductus arteriosus, when the fetal duct that diverts blood from the lungs fails to close; and ventricular and atrial septal defects, holes in the septum, the thin wall that divides the right and left sides of the heart. At the moment, there didn't seem to be any related symptoms, but it was an ominous find.

An eye exam at two days found that the baby did react to light, through closed lids. But there were multiple problems in the delicate structure of the eyes. The diagnosis was microphthalmos—abnormally small eyes—and opacified corneas, the normally clear layers of tissue through which light enters the eye. One of the chambers of the eyes was not formed, and a tear drainage system could not be found.

There was good news about one system, though. Close urological examination and then the results of genetic testing confirmed that this baby was the girl they had been expecting. Once again Kate and Paul shifted their thinking—their baby was Michaila, and it was a huge relief to post her name over her bed in the NICU. It was a relief, too, that there was no doubt about the gender. The baby had double-X chromosomes and female reproductive organs. The reason for the ambiguity was a surge of testosterone that had been produced shortly before birth, causing swelling of the external genitalia. John Gearhart, head of pediatric urology at Hopkins, assured the Disneys that the abnormality could be corrected with relatively simple cosmetic surgery.

But less optimistic news came when Michaila was eight days old, in a meeting with Rebecca Ichord, the pediatric neurologist who examined the baby's brain scans. By this time, Kate had been discharged from the hospital, and she and Paul were staying at the Children's House, a building across the street from the hospital where parents and families of children undergoing treatment can stay for a nominal fee. In the NICU conference room, with a group of interns, residents, and nurses listening, Dr. Ichord explained that Michaila's brain remained so compressed by excess cerebrospinal fluid that it was impossible to determine what was there. "Mr. and Mrs. Disney, we have to tell you, we've never seen this before," she said. "We can't tell you what this means, and we can't tell you what she will be capable of. We don't know if she'll ever walk or talk."

Kate and Paul chose to look upon this uncertain prognosis as good news. They felt it gave them hope that once the brain was decompressed, it would be normal.

Three days later, they decided to leave the immediate vicinity of the hospital for the first time since Michaila's birth. "We're going home to go to church," Paul told the NICU nurse. "Beep us if anything happens." There was some concern because the baby was breathing rapidly; a new device had been attached, nasal C-PAP, which pushed measured amounts of oxygen into the lungs through nasal prongs. But they knew Michaila was in good hands and they would be less than an hour away.

He is able
More than able
To conquer anything
That comes our way
To help us with what
Concerns us today

—*HE IS ABLE*, HYMN, PART OF PRAISING SERVICE

Hope

In the silence that followed the praising music at the Chesapeake Christian Fellowship, Paul's beeper went off. He and Kate quickly found a phone and called the NICU. "The baby is showing symptoms of heart failure, and it would be a good idea to get here as soon as you can," said a doctor. Within minutes, they were on the highway, speeding toward Baltimore, Paul going faster than one hundred miles per hour. Sitting next to him, Kate clenched her hands and felt pain in her own heart. *God, get us there safely, please let there be no police on this road. Lord, stabilize Michaila, help her through this crisis.*

In the NICU, Dr. Northington told them Michaila's heart was losing the strength it needed for pumping. She was in congestive heart failure, and if it hadn't already affected her liver and kidneys, it soon might. They would have to make a decision whether to put her back on a ventilator and other life supports. By the time Paul and Kate sat down to consider what they had to do, their parents had arrived at the hospital. Kate clutched her father's hands. "You need to pretend you're not my dad, just my pastor," she said. Paul prayed fervently for guidance and answers. *Lord, take this decision out of our hands, make our course apparent.* As Paul was saying "amen," Javier Repetto, a neonatology fellow, stuck his head in the room. "This may just be an infection and here's what we need to do," he said, authoritative and definitive, just the tone Kate was hoping for. "We can put her back on the vent, give her digoxin to help her heart pump, start her on antibiotics, see how she responds." Paul and Kate gave quick agreement to this plan, relieved that they did not have to make a decision about life supports. To all of the assembled family, it seemed they'd received an immediate answer from God to their request for an apparent course.

Michaila responded to the treatment, and two days later pulled out her own breathing tube. It is not unusual for infants to extubate themselves, and by then Michaila was breathing well enough on her own to do without the tube and the ventilator it was attached to. Kate was delighted that the baby had exercised her will. To her the message was clear: *I'm going to make it, I'll be fine.*

A week later, Paul and Kate took another break from the hospital and went to look for a gift for the baby in the Disney Store, in a downtown mall just minutes away. While they were away, Ben Carson decided to stop in the NICU and see how Michaila was doing. Shopping, Kate suddenly felt Paul squeeze her hand and pull her toward a phone. Once again they had been beeped. This time they hurried back to the hospital to find that Carson, who had delayed shunt surgery until the baby was stronger and more stable, was concerned about the feel of Michaila's head and some episodes of slow heart rate. It was time for the VP shunt to be installed, and Carson had rushed her into surgery. The shunt established a "good spontaneous flow," he wrote in his operative notes, and "the patient tolerated all of this quite well."

Once the shunt was in and the fluid draining, the MRIs showed her brain gradually expanding to fill the skull. Within two days the doctors could see enough to rule out the holoprosencephaly diagnosis—clearly, there were two well-defined hemispheres of Michaila's brain. However, Carson thought it looked like the corpus callosum, a bundle of nerve fibers between the two hemispheres, was missing. This structure is involved with information transfer between the hemispheres, and if it is impaired or missing, the results can be severe—or they can be mild or even asymptomatic.

By early November, Paul and Kate were focused on getting Michaila home. Whatever continuing medical attention the baby needed, her parents were convinced she would grow and develop better at home than in a hospital. Feeding was the major obstacle. Michaila's life had begun sustained by intravenous nourishment, and learning how to bottle-feed had been delayed by her surgeries. She wasn't sure what she was supposed to do with this rubber nipple being stuck in her mouth. Kate or Paul fed her, or tried, every three hours. The doctor had explained that infant feeding consisted of three functions: sucking, swallowing, and breathing, all at the same time. Kate prayed as she sat with Michaila in her arms in the NICU and tried to get her to take the bottle, *Please God, allow Michaila to suck, swallow, and breathe.*

If she didn't start eating, she would need a stomach tube, the doctors warned, but in another week Michaila was taking the bottle well enough to be discharged from the hospital. She came home to the little blue house in Edgewater on her due date, November 11, and did well. Days became somewhat more predictable. Paul was able to stop taking so much time off work. But even though each day no longer brought a crisis, the Disneys were learning what life was like with a medically fragile child. In early December, Kate felt two lumps in Michaila's abdomen, and the baby was diagnosed with an inguinal hernia, a piece of her intestine popping into her abdominal cavity. This is seen frequently in premature babies, and John Gearhart did the routine surgical repair at Hopkins. The next month she needed another operation to correct the flow speed of the shunt, and Ben Carson took care of that.

Around Christmas, Paul began to act uncharacteristically cranky. He had other symptoms, also—he felt thirsty and had to urinate frequently. He couldn't fail to recognize them—both his father and brother had type 1 diabetes, the form of the disease that usually strikes in childhood or adolescence and requires lifelong insulin injections. Paul was twenty-one and thought he'd escaped. But a blood glucose test confirmed his self-diagnosis, and he began the injections and dietary modifications that would be part of the rest of his life.

Meanwhile, Michaila was gaining weight, although feeding remained a struggle. Everyone was giving Kate "new mom" advice, and sometimes it was hard for her to hold on to her patience and not scream, "My baby isn't like other babies!" It was unclear how much Michaila could see or hear, but she did seem to have some light and sound perception. After a clinic visit with Ben Carson on December 30, he wrote in her chart, "She is very bright and alert, looks around, tracks objects, and turns toward sound. She has started to smile . . .

Overall Michaila is progressing and developing very well, with dramatic decreases in fluid spaces in her head."

In January, when Michaila was three months old, Jose Camacho, the geneticist who was trying to determine if there was a genetic cause of her collection of disabilities, came up with an answer. The nature of her abnormalities led him to focus on a portion of the X chromosome designated as Xp22.31. Discovery of an abnormality in Michaila's DNA in precisely this location confirmed the diagnosis of a rare syndrome called MIDAS, an acronym for microphthalmia (small eyes), dermal aplasia (skin disorder), and sclerocornea (hard cornea). It is also referred to as MLS, for microphthalmia with linear skin defects. First described in the medical literature in 1990, it affected only females; it was believed it would be lethal to a male fetus.

Camacho told Paul and Kate that only sixteen cases of MIDAS syndrome had been written up worldwide, and only two in the United States before Michaila. He told them that because it was so rare, it was difficult to predict how Michaila would do. The documented cases had a range of severity. Some of the girls had died in infancy. Many had some of the same features as Michaila, such as heart defects and genital anomalies.

To Paul and Kate, the way Camacho presented the diagnosis was encouraging and positive. "Not everything about a syndrome applies to everyone who has it," he said. "Michaila will be what Michaila will be, regardless of what this syndrome implies. We look at the child, not the syndrome."

~

Thank You, Lord, for our daughter, Michaila. Please, Lord, let it be in Your will to allow her to see Your wonders and to hear the beauty of Your works. Strengthen both her and us to handle everything put before us. We pray that You will be glorified through all of this.

In February 1997, when Michaila was five months old, a team of ophthalmologists attempted a corneal transplant of her left eye, the eye where the doctors thought there was the best chance of success. Eye exams indicated that she did have some light perception, but once surgery had begun and they were actually in the eye, the doctors could see that the abnormalities were more severe and pervasive than they had suspected. Intraocular pressure was elevated—glaucoma—and the retina was totally detached. The retina is the thin layer of transparent tissue at the back of the eye containing the rods and cones, the light-sensing cells. In a healthy eye, it is attached to the back wall of the sphere of the eye; vision cannot occur if it is detached. Eugene deJuan, Jr., an expert in retinal attachment, was called to the operating room, and he repaired the detachment. A cornea was transplanted. But the eye doctors told Paul and Kate that possibilities for success were limited.

Two weeks later, Michaila developed an infection in her left eye, and the new cornea was rejected. It was a setback—to Paul and Kate it seemed that their little girl turned inward. She no longer played with the toys they put in her crib or playpen. Her interest didn't go further than her own fingers and toes. As always, they turned to prayer, and it was to prayer that they attributed Michaila's turnaround, because gradually she started reaching out again, exploring, examining toys with her fingers and toes, interacting with the touch of her parents, rolling from one end of her crib to the other.

During some of the medical visits, the Disneys found the professionals amazed by how Michaila reached for toys and responded to touch. Paul and Kate began to videotape her activities at home, accumulating documentation of her accomplishments. She was a cute baby, small for her age, behind age norms in development, but clearly moving forward. She loved to be picked up and tossed in the air and carried piggyback. Outside, she turned to the breeze and smiled as the wind touched her face. Her skin problems had resolved, leaving only a small red spot on her neck that looked like a birthmark. Her heart, too, had healed with medication and growth, and she wouldn't need heart surgery. No one was sure how much she could hear, and that would be evaluated in future exams. She faced urological surgery in the next years, but none of her problems were life threatening.

Call unto Me, and I will answer thee; and show thee great and mighty things, which thou knowest not.

—JEREMIAH 33:3

In April, Kate learned she was pregnant. She couldn't believe it, and at first was depressed. "How am I going to do all I have to do to help Michaila when I'm pregnant, and then with another baby?" she sighed to her mother, once again feeling overwhelmed. The answer to the question was, in fact, her mom; Dee Packett lived only five miles away, didn't work outside her home, and was able to provide backup care. Paul's parents, Dan and Laura Disney, were also close by and willing to help with Michaila.

They all worried that this baby might also have this dreadful syndrome, and were relieved when a sonogram in July showed the fetus was a boy. He was due January 1, 1998.

In August, Michaila was hospitalized for a week, when misdirected fluid from her shunt filled her lungs. During this hospitalization, Kate and Paul heard for the first time about the Christ statue under the dome. They packed Michaila and a buffer of pillows into a wagon from the pediatrics playroom, and headed for the elevator, and the statue. *Funny that it took us so long to see this,* Kate thought as she admired the marble figure. Whatever the reason, she was sure it was God's plan. She prayed:

Standing here, Lord, in front of this giant statue of You, reminds us of how big You truly are. Thank You, Lord, for being bigger than this crisis. We know that through Your strength we will persevere.

Kate's labor began on Labor Day, September 1. At twenty-two weeks, the baby would not have much chance of survival. She was put on terbutaline to stop the contractions, and they eased for a couple of days, then started gradually building. She managed to hold out for two more weeks, but Nathaniel was born on September 14, weighing one pound, twelve ounces. He spent three months in the neonatal intensive care unit at Anne Arundel Medical Center. For those months, Dee took care of Michaila, while Kate and Paul spent as much time as they could with the new baby. *Maybe I've been too protective,* Kate thought when Michaila began to crawl in that period, away from her watchful eye.

They brought Nathaniel home on December 5, and suddenly "family" had a different meaning. Michaila was no longer the baby, although even with the developmental delays of extreme prematurity, Nathaniel was soon passing his big sister in all of the childhood milestones—eating, walking, talking, and understanding.

Michaila's second year of life was punctuated with operations. She was fitted with eye prosthetics, soft plastic hemispheres with a concave inner surface that fit over her own small eyes. Michaila had enough of an iris for observers to tell that her eyes were blue, like her mother's, and so were the prosthetics, which moved with her own eyes and kept the bones of the face from drawing too close together. In April 1998, deJuan attempted a retinal attachment of the right eye, but it was unsuccessful. Again, the Disneys felt that Michaila lost ground after this, and became less responsive. In May, Gearhart and his associates corrected the urological problems—further surgery would be necessary, but this was a big step. "[T]he cosmetic result is superb," Gearhart wrote to Michaila's pediatrician in Annapolis. "She looks like a normal little girl . . . She can be in the swimming pool, shower, or whatever."

Through these operations and the recovery periods, Michaila remained good natured and smiley. She was so active in her hospital bed that she sometimes pulled out her IVs. Sometimes Kate would drive home after hearing a depressing progress report from a doctor, close to tears, and the sound of Michaila's laughter in the backseat would restore peace to her mind. From Michaila came a very special understanding of what a real hug is, a real smile, a real giggle. Paul and Kate couldn't—and didn't want to—imagine life without her.

The family paid a number of visits to The Divine Healer during Michaila's hospitalizations, and on May 25, 1998, recorded their prayer in the book in the rotunda:

> *Dear Lord,*
>
> *We want to thank You for Michaila. Thank You that she came out of her surgery well. Please touch her and give her strength. I know that You are the Divine Healer. Please give her sight. You have made the blind to see before—please do this with Michaila. Thy will be done!*
>
> *Love,*
> *Paul, Kate, Michaila &*
> *Nathaniel Disney*

Kate and Paul knew that Michaila was hearing impaired, but they weren't sure how impaired. In June 1998, when Michaila was a few months from her second birthday, she had a thorough hearing evaluation at Kennedy Krieger Institute, the pediatric rehabilitation hospital next door to Hopkins, which shares much of its professional staff with Hopkins. Testing indicated severe hearing impairment in both ears. Michaila had enough hearing to hear the roar of a truck engine only if she were right next to it. To her, a loud rock band would sound like a whisper.

She was fitted with hearing aids, and her world opened—a little. She could hear the baby crying, a vacuum cleaner, a slamming door, speech if the speaker was standing right next to her. Her own vocalization increased when the hearing aids were in and she babbled like a baby—like Nathaniel, in fact, who was beginning to make sounds and provided a useful role model for Michaila. But she soon plateaued with the hearing aids, and was still missing the majority of speech sounds that would allow her to understand and develop speech.

Eating continued to be a problem. Michaila's first teeth came in unevenly spaced and lacked sufficient enamel coating, and it hurt her to eat sweets. She liked salty foods—cheese crackers, hot dogs, grilled cheese sandwiches—but more often than not, she rejected food. This was one area in which Michaila had some control, Kate and Paul theorized, and her oral defensiveness was probably a reaction to having had tubes shoved down her throat so often in her young life. For the first time, they were dealing with a behavioral problem, not a physical problem, but it was potentially life threatening. In August 1998 Michaila was admitted to Hopkins for "failure to thrive," and fitted with a nasogastric tube, through her nose into her stomach, for feeding. The NG tube can be irritating and is usually a temporary solution. Three months later, the doctors installed a gastric tube directly into her stomach. It involved no discomfort and could remain in place for years. The formula dripped into the G tube four times a day would provide all the nutrition Michaila needed, until she was ready to eat real food.

The same month that Michaila got the G tube, Kate found out she was once again pregnant. Again it was unplanned and unexpected. Paul and Kate knew this would be their last child—they would take the necessary steps after this pregnancy to ensure that there would be no more. Meanwhile, Kate's was a high-risk pregnancy—she didn't want to have another premature birth. Examination found that her cervix probably couldn't hold the fetus in place, the reason Nathaniel had arrived so early. In February, her cervix was closed with a stitch, and she was ordered on bed rest for the remainder of the pregnancy. Again, both grandmothers filled the breech, taking care of Michaila and Nathaniel during the day, and Paul took over at night. It was another hard time, but it was worth it—Rachel was born June 5, 1999, the first Disney baby who had no problems, no NICU, no extended hospital stay. For the first time, Kate was able to enjoy the gratification of nursing. *What a different feeling this is, the way it's supposed to be,* she thought as she walked out of the hospital with her baby two days after the birth. She breathed a prayer of thanks:

> *Lord, I always dreamed of this day but I never thought it would happen. Thank You for helping me and my family get through this hard time. It was all worth it, staring into my beautiful daughter's eyes. Eyes that see and ears that hear. Oh, how much we take for granted. Help me to be a good mother to all of my children and never treat any of them different from the other.*

The three children grew and progressed and interacted—Kate and Paul could see that her younger siblings kept Michaila stimulated and moving forward, even though her pace was slower than theirs. That could be painful to watch—sometimes Kate felt she had to stifle her expectations for her firstborn and remind herself to accept what was given. But Michaila was active, able to roll on and off the couch, to pull herself up on furniture, to cruise around the living room holding on to things. She wasn't walking yet, but it would come soon. Paul and Kate tried to imagine what it would be like to not have sight and hearing as motivation, for example, to reach for an object or to let go of the couch and walk independently. *Not* having the senses we take for granted is very difficult to contemplate, even for the parents of a blind/hearing-impaired child.

Kate and Paul had heard about cochlear implants, a technology that goes beyond hearing aids to allow a hearing-impaired person to perceive sound. A miniature receiver with an array of electrodes is attached to the cochlea, a duct within the ear. Embedded in the skin behind the ear, the implant is magnetic, with an external microphone and transmitter attached to it. They are connected to a beeper-size processing unit, worn at the waist. The surgically implanted receiver approximates the missing sense with an electrical impulse to the brain. Children with these devices who have never had normal hearing now have the ability to perceive sound, but they must also receive intensive family support and speech therapy to make sense of the sound—to develop an understanding of language and learn to communicate with spoken language themselves.

Michaila received a cochlear implant in November 1999, in her left ear, the ear with the lesser hearing and further from the VP shunt. John Niparko, an otolaryngologist who came to Hopkins in 1991 to establish a cochlear implant program for children, rubbed the toe of The Divine Healer on the morning he operated on Michaila—he often does on surgery days. The procedure was complicated somewhat by slight malformations within Michaila's ear, but he was able to place the implant successfully. Niparko is one of the country's most experienced surgeons with cochlear implants. When he came to Hopkins, such procedures were just beginning, and he did about half a dozen a year. By the time Michaila received hers, he was performing more than one hundred cochlear implant procedures a year.

Activation of Michaila's implant was delayed a month, so she could recover from the surgery, and then the device was turned on slowly. By the new year, Paul and Kate were excited by clear evidence that Michaila's hearing was much improved—she tuned into her surroundings more than she had ever done before, laughed when she heard the laughter of her brother or sister or parents, and babbled new sounds, including "Mama." Her balance and equilibrium also stabilized, and she became more physically active, motivating her little body to where she wanted it to be with great energy. More than ever, her parents could see her stubborn and independent streak and her intelligence. Niparko agreed. "She showed progress very early on," he told Paul and Kate. "She was telling us that her brain is hungry for this information, and she's likely to be able to use it to develop that very complex behavior we know as speech and communication."

What is the future for Michaila Disney? In the twentieth century, Helen Keller proved to the world that there was no limit for a blind/hearing-impaired person. In the twenty-first, Michaila has the advantage of technology and medical advances that seemed science-fiction just decades ago. While the technology does not currently exist to give her sight, her optic nerve is intact, and ongoing scientific investigations promise to lead to a device that could one day allow her to see.

Full of respect for technology and their doctors and all the people who have helped Michaila get to where she is today, Paul and Kate Disney feel that a force greater than science has inspired their daughter's life. Their faith, and the God it connects them to, is behind everything, they are sure. It is in this faith that they find reasons for the way their lives have unfolded so far, and they thank God every day for the privilege of raising Michaila.

And we know that all things work together for good to them that love God, to them who are called according to His purpose.

—ROMANS 8:28

PATRICIA FOSARELLI
Renewal of Faith

Jesus, Son of God, have mercy on me as a sinner. Je-sus, Je-sus, Je-sus.

—THE JESUS PRAYER, OFTEN SHORTENED TO JUST THE TWO SYLLABLES, JE-SUS, AND KNOWN AS THE BREATHING PRAYER.

Patricia Fosarelli heard a call to become a physician and care for sick children when she was only twelve. There was no vision, no ringing bells, but a summons nonetheless, clear as a clarion: that she was meant to spend her life as a pediatrician.

No, not a nurse, she insisted, when her parents, both born to Italian immigrants, asked why not nursing rather than medicine. But Pat was so bright and focused and competent that they were totally supportive. She was an only child, and Margie and Del Fosarelli doted on her.

She was a thoughtful but happy girl, with an avid curiosity about the world and a steadfast faith in God. As a toddler, she took her toys apart to try to figure out how they worked. She was reading before she started school and once in school, she read voraciously, from the books she was assigned in her Catholic school classrooms to the variety of materials in the public library. In school, her reading speed was clocked at over one thousand words per minute, more than five times the average. She sometimes ripped through a book or more a day.

She nurtured her faith at church on Sundays and throughout the week, seeing God in nature, in the love of her parents, in the feeling of community in her neighborhood, a working-class suburb just east of Baltimore. From her earliest memories, Pat felt the presence of God and Jesus in her life. She was the kid who liked church, who never tried to get out of it. When she was a young child, she would swing on a swing in her backyard and literally breathe her prayer, just the simple name of Jesus. *Je-* ascending and inhaling on the syllable; *sus-* coming down and exhaling. *Je-sus, Je-sus, Je-sus*—it was comfort and sustenance for her. She felt the wind through her hair as she swung, and the thought that God was playing with her hair brought a smile to her face and more meaning to the prayer. *Je-sus, Je-sus, Je-sus.*

When she was older and saw herself as a pediatrician, she never doubted that this was God's plan for her. She stayed focused on her goal. She was an A student at the Catholic High School of Maryland, graduating in 1969, and the yearbook noted her career plan. In her spare time she volunteered at City Hospitals (now Johns Hopkins Bayview Medical Center) and across town at a clinic in west Baltimore. At the College of Notre Dame of Maryland, she majored in chemistry. She was accepted at the University of Maryland Medical School, in downtown Baltimore. She lived at home, and for the short commute her parents bought her a Dodge Dart, the first car the family had ever owned, since neither of her parents drove.

So tenderly You
unfold me, then enfold me
into holy You. *

Medical school and her internship and residency were a revelation. The long and grueling hours, the frenetic pace, the lack of time for sleep—that was one element, a physical draining that Pat had never

* The haiku in this chapter are by Patricia Fosarelli.

before experienced. She felt tired all the time. But even more intense was the emotional impact of some of the things she saw: a toddler in the emergency room with head injuries and broken bones that came from being thrown against a wall. Neglected children, unfed and unwashed and unloved. A boy with a malignant brain tumor, doomed to die young. Teenage drug addicts with not much more promising a future than children with deadly cancers. There seemed no end to the misery and pain.

Pat was confused and troubled. *Wait a minute,* she said to herself, *I thought the good were rewarded for being good. These poor kids never hurt anyone. Why are they suffering so much?* It didn't seem consistent with the compassionate God who had tousled her hair on the swing. She realized what a sheltered life she had led, surrounded by love and faith. In the context of her religious upbringing, she could make no sense of the children she saw in this inner city hospital. Her own faith had always been a big part of what held her together. Now it seemed useless. She felt helpless in the face of the burden of the kids she saw.

> *Young children starving*
> *in a nation overfed—*
> *more obscene than porn.*

She was so saddened by her experiences that for the first time in her life, she didn't want to go to church. She didn't want to pray. Her churchgoing dwindled to every couple of weeks, to less than once a month, to just Christmas and Easter, to not at all. Her parents were upset. This was a rejection of their life's work in raising her. "If this is the cost of being a doctor, it's not worth it," her mother declared. "I just don't get anything from the Mass anymore," Pat told her. "It's a waste of time for me to go."

"Why are you warring with God?" her father wanted to know. "I'm not," Pat answered. "I don't even know if God exists."

One of the cases that would always stay with her was a ten-year-old boy with a brain tumor. She was an intern at University Hospital, and the boy, who was her patient, had a poor prognosis. But his family was convinced if they prayed hard enough, he would get better. Pat watched them pray and it seemed futile. Even worse, she felt that because of their faith that he would recover with prayer alone, they were increasing and prolonging his suffering by neglecting treatment that might give him some relief. The medical team urged the parents to accept some of the treatments, but they refused. When he was discharged, the hospital lost track of him, but a year later he came back into the hospital in grave condition and soon lapsed into a coma. The child died within several days. Pat was a resident on the boy's unit, and she felt her disillusion deepen as she watched him die.

Another experience touched her in a different way. In her senior year of medical school, a rotation in internal medicine took her to the Veterans Administration Hospital. She was the student doctor of a man with advanced liver disease, a sweet, undemanding patient who told her stories of his life and the alcoholism that had ravaged him. Everyone liked him, and when the cardiac arrest bells went off one Saturday evening as most of the staff was eating, they left their food and rushed to his room.

Resuscitation had already begun when Pat got there, and the effort was intense—a series of increasingly more powerful shocks with defibrillator paddles, then injections of epinephrine and lidocaine into his IV line, to stimulate his heart chemically. The struggle to bring him back continued for more than a half hour, a long time for someone's heart to be stopped, but with the team breathing for him through a bag over his mouth and nose, and with manual chest compressions, the patient's heart finally started on its own. The assembled medical staff broke into spontaneous applause.

The man came to consciousness with a dazed look on his face. He fixed his glassy eyes on Pat, and said, "I thought you liked me."

"I do," she answered quickly.

"Then why didn't you let me stay where I was?"

"Where were you?"

He didn't answer right away. Then he said in a sad voice, "I just want to go back to the light, the light that loved me." He repeated again and again, "The light loved me."

"What light?" Pat asked.

"*The* light," he insisted.

This was years before books and TV shows publicized numerous near-death experiences in which people perceived a bright, welcoming light as they passed away. Neither Pat nor her colleagues had ever heard of what this man was talking about. Later that night, he pulled out his IV lines and was put in restraints. He begged Pat to discontinue his treatment and let him "go back to the light."

Pat was moved in a way she had never felt before for a patient. She went home and sobbed. The man died the next day, and she felt a sense of mournful relief for him, but it was years before she thought of his bright light in the context of the spiritual or the divine. At that point in her life, that wasn't the way she was thinking.

Even as her faith in God wavered, Pat was still devoted to being a pediatrician. She no longer saw her calling in spiritual terms, but taking care of sick and hurt kids remained an ethical imperative for her. When she finished her residency, she accepted a Robert Wood Johnson fellowship in general academic pediatrics at The Johns Hopkins Hospital. It was a great honor, and she was excited about the opportunities it provided to work in the clinic and do research. She was also looking forward to a more normal schedule and a little more sleep in her life. She felt upbeat and positive the first time she walked through the Broadway lobby and encountered The Divine Healer. Even though she'd grown up in Baltimore, she'd never seen the statue before.

She was stunned by the towering marble sculpture. *Yo, baby, what is this I'm seeing?* she asked herself as she walked around the base and admired the cool gray artistry of the work. Agnostic as she had become, there was no erasing the images of her childhood and teenage years, the importance Christ once had in her life. She felt awed by the statue, and glad she was going to be working in the hospital where it stood.

I open my arms
hoping to embrace You, but
sensing You, I flee.

Catherine DeAngelis, then director of the division of general pediatrics and adolescent medicine, was Pat's fellowship director at Hopkins. Like Pat, she was a Roman Catholic, raised in the church, educated at Catholic schools. Unlike Pat, she had never lost her faith, although she, too, was disturbed by the suffering she saw treating children in the inner city. Cathy knew Pat had grown up in the church, but suspected that her churchgoing had lapsed.

"Where do you go to church, Fos?" Cathy asked one day.

Pat could only stutter. "Uh . . . uh . . . Why do you ask?"

"A good Catholic girl like you should be going to church."

"I don't want to talk about it."

But Cathy DeAngelis wouldn't let it go. Pat brushed off her admonitions, but Cathy persisted. As the mentoring relationship evolved into friendship, Cathy sensed a need that was not being met for her younger colleague, something missing in Pat's life. Ever the activist, she decided to force the issue. Pat was visiting her home one Saturday afternoon and Cathy suggested, "Let's go get a video."

When they got in the car, though, Cathy didn't go to the video store. She pulled up in front of Saints Philip and James Church in north Baltimore. Pat looked at her warily. "What's this all about?"

"Oh, didn't I tell you? I always go to church on Saturday afternoons," Cathy said breezily.

Pat was furious. "You tricked me," she said accusingly.

"You can just wait in the car if you want," Cathy said.

Pat thought about doing just that. She hadn't been in a church in nine years and had not been thinking about going back. But she was in an unfamiliar neighborhood and didn't know if she was safe. She followed Cathy up the steps and into the back of the church, plastered herself into the last pew and said to herself, *I'm staying right here.* Her thought flew out to a God she didn't know if she believed in. *You got me here but I am not moving forward.*

But an inroad had been made, her dormant spirituality tweaked. Even from the back pew, Pat felt a faint rekindling of what had been such an important part of her youth. In the months that followed, she found herself at church more and more frequently, first with Cathy, then on her own. It felt like coming home and filled a void she had worked hard to ignore.

> *You duped me, Lord, and I let myself be duped. You were too strong for me, and You triumphed. . . . I said to myself, I will not mention God, I will speak God's name no more. But then it becomes like a fire burning in my heart, imprisoned in my bones. I grow weary holding it in, I cannot endure it.*
>
> —JEREMIAH 20:7, 9

Pat finished the fellowship in 1983, when she was thirty, left for another job in Virginia but soon came back to a position at Hopkins. As it turned out, her father was ill at the time. It was cancer, and by the time the surgeons opened him up, it had spread too widely to tell where it originated.

Del Fosarelli died three weeks after Pat's return to Baltimore, in 1983, and Pat and her mother clung to each other in their grief. Margie had eleven brothers and sisters, Del had four, so there was plenty of family to share in the mourning. Pat wished she could get the comfort most of her family got from their religion, but for her something was still lacking.

Nevertheless, there had been a shift. As Pat's spirituality reawakened, it affected her work in the clinic. Now she had a new context for questions like "Dr. Pat, does God want me to be sick?" or "Why did my mommy die, Dr. Pat?" She felt her faith helped her to be a better doctor. Her patients' parents, she observed, often prayed, and she gained a better understanding of them through their prayers.

Through her thirties, she was doing exactly what she wanted to do, serving the medical needs of underprivileged youngsters. She studied and published articles about latchkey kids, and how telephone call-in services can help them; about the impact of television on children; about infectious diseases among inner city children in daycare settings. With another Hopkins pediatrician, Beryl Rosenstein, she co-authored *Pediatric Pearls,* a practical clinical handbook for pediatricians published in 1989. But then she started feeling restless and wanted to use her abilities to reach more children than those she could see in the clinic. She experienced health problems herself, felt puzzled and hurt at the way her body had betrayed her, but learned firsthand that she had the resources to fight back.

Pat tried a job change in 1992, taking the position of director of school health for the Baltimore City Health Department. She kept up her clinical skills as school doctor at the Baer School, for physically and emotionally challenged children. From 1993 to 1998, she also volunteered at the Shepherd's Clinic, a medical center for those without health insurance. But health department work was primarily administrative and not giving her the satisfaction she wanted. After four years, she was ready to move back into full-time clinical work. In 1996, Hopkins offered her a job as a physician in the Intensive Primary Care Pediatric Clinic, and she eagerly accepted.

The IPC treats high-risk inner city children with a variety of health concerns, and provides well-child and routine preventive care. Many of the children seen at the clinic are born to mothers with HIV disease, although most do not go on to develop HIV infection themselves. Pat was immediately drawn to the neediness of these children and families, not just medical need, but social and emotional as well. She was happy she could facilitate social services and follow families to make sure they continued getting help when necessary.

Meanwhile, Pat's continuing involvement with church and her renewed spirituality helped make sense of the medical work for her. In the late 1980s, she had moved forward from the back pew. "Can you read for us?" the pastor at Saints Philip and James asked her after the service one Sunday, and soon she moved to the lectern, reading scripture at Mass. Reading scripture to the congregation was a gratifying experience, the feeling of the word of God coming through her. But here, too, something was missing, and Pat wasn't sure what. As always in her life, she sought broader understandings, and she was still falling short of finding them.

Her pastor startled her one day by telling her, "I think it's time for you to get more theological education."

"I had sixteen years of theological education in Catholic schools," Pat retorted. "I think that's more than the national average. Anyway, I vowed never to enter a classroom again after medical school."

But the thought was planted and wouldn't go away. Some of her medical colleagues suggested that her brain might turn to mush if she pursued the "soft" study of theology, as opposed to hard science. Pat thought not. More and more, she was intrigued with the possibility of seeking answers in another context, of combining faith and medicine, looking for where the two could comfortably intersect.

Sometimes she was afraid she had missed a calling. Even before she wanted to be a doctor, like many devout Catholic girls she had flirted with the idea of being a nun. She had decided the convent was not for her but now and again wondered if it had been a correct decision. Once she started theological studies, she was convinced the dual track she had chosen—medicine and theology—was the way for her to best use the right and left sides of her brain, the science and the spirit.

Hope

Suspended in love
I am weightless, unfettered
By earth's gravity

In 1992, Pat began taking classes at the Ecumenical Institute of Theology, the evening division of Saint Mary's Seminary and University, in Baltimore, which offers master's level courses in theology. Working during the day, taking classes at night, and continuing with an active role at her church could be exhausting, but she was joyfully stimulated by the theological education. She got a master's degree in theology from the Institute in 1994, the most advanced degree it offered. The connection between the healing she did as a doctor and the faith she felt in God was clear to her, but she knew many of her colleagues were not convinced. *I need more credentials to convince them,* she thought determinedly. *If I'm going to have credibility in bringing together the physical, emotional, and spiritual, I'll need an advanced degree.* She enrolled in the doctorate program at Wesley Theological Seminary in Washington, D.C., writing her thesis on the spiritual development of children and earning a doctorate in ministry in 1997.

Michael Gorman, dean of the Ecumenical Institute, saw a combination of qualities in Pat that he was sure would be valuable to the Institute. To him she represented the integration of mind, body, and spirit, a holistic understanding of human beings that few could grasp with the sophistication of this physician/theologian. He was impressed by her ability to communicate the importance of the spirit to her medical colleagues and to emphasize the value of the body as well as the soul to her theological associates. He invited her to teach at the Ecumenical Institute in 1995 and appointed her as his assistant for church, community, and alumni relations. She crafted a course in health, disease, and spirituality and began teaching that; soon she expanded her role at the Institute by participating in a program in parish nursing, a growing movement nationwide. Gorman thought she was a living example to her students and the religious community that science and faith do not have to be at odds with each other.

Pat loved teaching, both at the Ecumenical Institute and the Hopkins School of Medicine. She felt relaxed and comfortable in front of a classroom. In developing a curriculum about medicine and spirituality, she applied the critical thinking she had developed in medicine to the ongoing academic effort to prove the connection between faith and healing. "It's difficult to tease out," she told a recent class at the Ecumenical Institute. She outlined the progression of studies, from reports that churchgoers had better health than nonchurchgoers to the application of prayer to specific diseases. She warned of the difficulty of proving cause and effect and the danger of drawing conclusions before study results are repeated. "Our information about this is in its infancy," she told her students, a class of about twenty that included healthcare professionals, clergy, and lay people. "Up to a few years ago, no one wanted to talk about this stuff. From 1970 to the mid-eighties there were less than a dozen articles in the *Index Medicus* related to spirituality and health. That's pathetic."

She continued teaching, turning to the physiological changes associated with expression of spirituality and how mental states induced by meditation or religious worship or the social support of a religious community can contribute to good health. "In the language of spirituality, this is all about an integrated life. You are who you are, no matter where you are. The goal of a life is to integrate, to be one person in all places."

She ended the class with a prayer: *Good and gracious God, we have no idea of how marvelous You are, and how marvelous we are. Open our eyes, our ears, our hearts so we can begin to understand this.*

⌇

Teaching, treating needy children, being part of her church—in her late forties, Pat felt she hadn't had such a good time since she was a teenager. Her joy in her work translated to excellent performance.

She had won teaching awards in both medicine and theology. The Central Maryland Ecumenical Council awarded her its Christian Life Award for the way she combined medicine, teaching, and theology.

The right and left sides of her brain were working together in other aspects of her life as well. She began talking to groups about her experiences and the path she had taken, and became increasingly in demand as a speaker before church and other groups. She hardly had time for hobbies—but managed to pursue interests in calligraphy and writing poetry. Much of her poetry was in the form of haiku and often expressed her spirituality. She found the succinct, simple format an ideal framework for her prayers.

Holy Arsonist
ablazed me. Sweet inferno
within and without.

Academic spirituality was not the only spirituality in Pat's life. After twelve years at Saints Philip and James, in 1992 she moved to Corpus Christi, a Baltimore church closer to downtown. There she met Sister Jane Coyle, pastoral director of the church. A pastoral director leads a congregation that has no resident priest and it is uncommon for a woman to hold the position. Sister Jane had been at Corpus Christi since 1980, and she was immediately impressed with Pat's energy and her generosity. Pat joined the church's liturgy (worship) committee, and moved on to chair this important group that planned the services.

Sister Jane was a member of the Medical Mission Sisters, an order that performs medically oriented work, primarily in developing countries. Pat gravitated to this gentle but compelling woman who had devoted her life to the same integration of spirit and body that Pat was exploring. She was attracted to the order's mission of holistic healing and in fall 1999 was accepted as a lay associate in the order.

In the IPC clinic one morning, the foster mother of a baby who had been exposed to HIV through his mother's drug use in pregnancy sat and rocked the baby in her arms while Pat was entering her notations on the patient's chart. *God loves you, God loves you, God loves you,* the woman crooned to the baby. Pat looked up and smiled, and the woman looked away in embarrassment. "Oh, I shouldn't have said that."

"Why not?" Pat asked.

"I thought you people don't believe in God," the woman said.

You people? Pat wondered. She guessed the woman was talking about doctors. "Some of us certainly do believe in God," she reassured the woman. She didn't know how the families she treated, many with so few resources and such huge problems, could survive *without* faith.

During another recent day at the clinic, she had to call upon her own faith for solace, to seek sense of the pain and unfairness she saw around her. In the morning, a seventeen-year-old girl who had been hospitalized with AIDS died of the disease. She had been seen at the clinic longer than anyone else, something of a miracle because she had been infected at birth through her mother, but lived most of her life disease free. But her last years had been filled with painful infections and progressive debilitation. Her caretakers were her grandparents, and neither of them could make it to the hospital as she lay dying. The previous month, the girl had asked not to be left alone as her end neared, and Pat was with her as she drew her last breaths. It seemed so cruel that this girl who had conquered so much adversity finally lost her battle.

For the rest of the day, Pat kept thinking she wanted to go home, that she didn't have the emotional fortitude to continue examining babies and children and keeping up a cheerful dialogue with their parents. But, of course, she stayed. Alone in her office for a few minutes, she started crying, recovered, and found herself crying again an hour later. *What a tragedy, how this girl suffered,* she thought. Finally, at the end of her day she walked out through the Broadway lobby, in search of fresh outdoor air to lift her spirits. She wasn't thinking about the statue, but there He was as she walked around the staircase. His presence suffused the lobby. She had grown to love the spirit the statue engendered, how people became gentler and more vulnerable as they stood and prayed there. She looked at The Divine Healer with a feeling of profound sadness. *Why does something as bad as this have to happen to a child?* It seemed an unanswerable question. She turned and left the building, still with sadness, but now with a feeling of peace from being in the presence of the statue. He inspired her own prayer:

> *God, thanks for Laura—*
> *She taught me about living*
> *as she lay dying.*

As she walked to her car, her thoughts shifted from Laura's death to her life, and she found her mind filled with the always comforting breathing prayer, a syllable for each step she took: *Je-sus, Je-sus, Je-sus.*

> *You—Source, Guide, and Goal*
> *Embarking Point, Journey, and*
> *Destination—You.*

Part Two

CONSOLATION

THE CANFIELD/PARKER TWINS
Young Souls

God, please give us strength, please give us hope.
Please, God, help us through these hard times,
help Vanessa hang on, help her give birth to
healthy babies.

—RICHARD PARKER, JULY 1998

Vanessa Canfield felt she had prayed for things all her life and God had hardly ever delivered. Prayers seemed a waste of time anyway, at least for her in her short but tough life. She wasn't even sure she believed in God. She couldn't see Him. How could she believe in what she couldn't see? In fact, sometimes it seemed that God was dead-set against her. She'd known rejection, she'd known abuse, she'd known violence, she'd known neglect, she'd known pain. And now she was twenty-one, on the verge of doing what she wanted most, becoming a mother. She was pregnant with twins, and God—if He existed at all—was making it harder for her than she would have thought possible.

Richard Parker, the twins' father, was five years older than Vanessa and had known trouble his whole life too. But now, with Vanessa having so much difficulty with her pregnancy, his thinking and faith were going the opposite direction from hers. *Somebody, some force has to be there to run this crazy world,* he thought. His prayers seemed to flow in a constant stream as Vanessa lay in a hospital bed through July and early August 1998, and they waited for their babies to be born. One day, wandering around the hospital, he followed a group of people into the administration building, walked around the corner and was amazed to see the Jesus statue. *This thing is huge!* he marveled. He walked around to the front and stood in awe. Finally, here was a recipient for his free-floating prayers. A warm feeling coursed through him and he remained for fifteen minutes, more comforted than he had ever before felt in his life.

~

They hadn't even known each other a year yet. Rick was a friend of Vanessa's brother Troy. Rick and Troy lived in Hagerstown, a town of about 37,000 nestled in the foothills of the Appalachian Mountains in western Maryland, where one of the biggest employers is a Mack Truck factory. Vanessa had lived in Hagerstown until she was thirteen. She got in trouble early. Smoking cigarettes when she was six, getting dizzy when she was only eight from drinking the airline miniatures of booze that her mother always had around. Looking back, she saw herself as a hellion who would do "ornery" things just to get attention. Once in elementary school, when a boy was being disrespectful to the girls, she punched him. That got her to the principal's office, where the principal beat her with a paddle. When she went home and her mother saw the welts, she raised hell with the school.

But Vanessa's mom could be abuser as well as protector, and put some welts of her own on the girl. Her dad wasn't in the picture; he had left when she was two, and Vanessa never saw him. She was a tomboy who liked to play football with the boys—until she began to grow breasts and found out how much it could hurt to be tackled. By then she was starting to think girlish thoughts—like what it would feel like to kiss a boy.

When she was eleven, she ended up in foster care. She hated it. She kept running away and over the next couple of years was in three different homes, three different middle schools. Obviously, foster care wasn't the solution for this impulsive and sometimes reckless girl. When she was thirteen, Vanessa left Hagerstown to live with her grandmother in Cleveland.

It was a good move. She got along much better with her grandmother than she had with her mother and the various foster parents and settled down a little in her high school years. But she was still impetuous and impertinent, and flouted most of the rules and boundaries she confronted. In 1997, she came back to Hagerstown for a visit with her mother and brother, and Troy told her he didn't like the life she was leading. Why not come back to Hagerstown and try living with their mother again? Now that she was twenty, almost an adult herself, maybe things would be smoother.

Vanessa decided to move back. Troy took her around and introduced her to some of his friends. One afternoon, they stopped at Richard Parker's house. Rick was there with two young children, and Vanessa wasn't sure what the story was. Rick acted like a dad, but there didn't seem to be a wife. Later Troy told her they were Rick's children but was vague about his friend's marital status and didn't know where the mother was, though the children spent most of their time with her.

Vanessa was tremendously taken with this tall (six feet, six inches!), good-looking young man. She liked his tattoos—she had a few of her own, but nothing to match the more than thirty that he had all over his body. She liked his smile and the way he was with his kids. When he was talking to her, she suddenly felt uncharacteristically shy, and stuttered out a "no" when on their first meeting he asked her if she wanted something to drink.

While Vanessa sat and talked to the children, Troy and Rick stepped away into the laundry room. Rick wanted to find out more about this pretty little sister. Mainly, did she have a boyfriend? No, Troy said, she had just moved back to town. They were going to a party that night and Rick invited himself along.

Vanessa floated out of Rick's house and felt buoyant with excitement. She wondered what Rick would think if he knew what she was feeling. *Be careful,* she said to herself, *you don't want him to think you're fast and easy. Better hold it in for a while.* After she left, Rick sat down to a video game and when he had to enter a name, he unconsciously typed in "Vanessa." *Whoa, what am I doing?* he thought. *She's way too pretty for me.*

Rick was born in Pensacola, Florida. His father, married to someone else, walked out on his mother when she became pregnant. His mother abandoned him when he was two days old, left him in the care of a friend. This friend was the person Rick called Mom. He didn't pursue any contact with his biological mother, but did finally meet his biological father when he was twenty-one. But it was Claude and Linda Parker whom he considered his parents. They moved to Hagerstown when he was five.

Rick grew up with a determination not to live his life regretting his childhood. His own marriage hadn't been good, but he had tried. Tried so hard he ended up in jail, after starting a fight with someone who said bad things about his wife. He was convicted of assault and did three weeks in the local jail, only to find when he came out that his wife had used the time to start seeing someone else. The marriage was doomed—as soon as they could pull the money together, they'd get divorced, though that hadn't happened yet. But he loved his kids and stayed involved with them. As part of the terms of his probation, he took a parenting course from the county department of social services, and was named "father of the year." But there was now no woman in his life.

At the party the night they met, Vanessa thought it would have been awfully boring if Rick hadn't been there. He turned out to have a good singing voice and interacted with everyone, seemed to be everyone's friend. Over the next couple of weeks she saw him three or four times, when he was with her brother. Then one night he came over to her mother's and they listened to music together. He liked country music, she liked heavy metal, but their differences didn't seem to matter. They started spending more time with each other. It was December and they got a Christmas tree together. After Christmas, he came over one morning and it snowed all day. Outside, fooling around in the snow, throwing snowballs, Vanessa's younger sister came up to Rick and asked in a bratty little-sister way, "When are you going to kiss her?"

This is going to be in my time. I'm going to do this right, Rick thought. *I don't want to screw things up.* Later, he and Vanessa were standing under a tree and she started shivering. "I'm cold too," Rick said, and Vanessa pulled his hands under her arms to warm them. Rick kissed her, a long sweet kiss with promise of a future. He had to bend down more than a foot to do it, and they laughed about that. *Wow,* Vanessa thought, *it's December but it feels like the Fourth of July.*

~

Vanessa couldn't believe how attracted she was to Rick and how mutual it seemed to be. As a teenager, she'd had some relationships that hadn't been great, and this was a lot different. This felt like what she'd been waiting for. She already knew she was in love with Rick by the time she found out he had a wife. She wasn't crazy about that, but trusted him that the divorce would happen when there was some extra money. Rick had a job as a carpenter and was a steady, dependable worker. Soon they were spending every night together. Intimacy came quickly and easily—they felt comfortable and right together. *She's a handful,* Rick thought, *but I've got big hands. I can take care of her.*

According to her calculation, Vanessa became pregnant in late January or early February. "I wouldn't mind having your baby," she told Rick in February when her period was late. She saw the fear in his eyes then. A month later the pregnancy was confirmed by a test at a local women's health clinic. They walked out hand in hand. "How do you feel about this?" Vanessa asked Rick. He squeezed her hand.

"You know I love you and I love kids," he answered. "I'm excited, but I have to admit I'm scared."

The day of the positive pregnancy test was Friday, March 13, and in the months to come Rick and Vanessa would look back and see the warning of bad luck foretold by that date. By mid-April she was feeling crampy, with a lot of pressure in her lower back. It was severe enough so that she went to the hospital emergency room late one night, and ended up being admitted to the maternity unit of Washington County Hospital. In the morning, the doctors would do an ultrasound and have the results of the cultures they had taken, and maybe an explanation for why her uterus seemed to be bigger than it should be at this early stage of pregnancy.

Rick spent the night in the hospital with Vanessa, and was only half awake at seven-thirty A.M. when the nurse wheeled in the ultrasound apparatus and started moving the wand over Vanessa's still flat abdomen. She could see the wavering lines on the screen, like two little circles. *That's not the way it's supposed to look,* she thought fearfully, but the nurse turned to her with a grin. "You've got twins," she said. "That explains why your uterus is farther along than we would have expected." Vanessa was delighted. Now that she knew what she was looking at, the ultrasound image of the babies looked like two cute little frogs. She was still having cramps, but those sensations were overpowered by the happy knowledge that she was carrying twins. She got a printout of the sonogram so they could show the first "picture" of the babies to their friends and family. She left the hospital that afternoon.

She was put on terbutaline, a muscle relaxant, to ease her cramping. The cramping became intermittent, then went away altogether. Things went smoothly for the next couple of months. Vanessa was seeing Eva Olah, a Hagerstown obstetrician, and seemed to be on course. Her belly was growing and she started to feel the babies move. Rick and Vanessa dared relax and let themselves think everything would be okay. From the sonogram, they knew both babies were boys. They named them—one was Troy, for Vanessa's brother, who had introduced them; the other was Travis, for Rick's favorite country singer, Travis Tritt. Both twins had the same middle name: Allen, for Rick's middle name.

Vanessa had a little bit of a bloody discharge in early July, but there were no contractions and the doctor said she seemed to be fine. Then one night in mid-July, she woke up feeling wet between her legs. She wanted to believe she was leaking urine, but she knew it wasn't urine—the fluid felt thick and syrupy. *Trouble again,* she thought. In the emergency room she got into an argument with the midwife who examined her. The midwife insisted the fluid was urine. "Look, lady, I know the difference," snapped Vanessa, exasperated and frightened. "I've been peeing for twenty-one years now, I know where it comes from and what it feels like."

A test showed she was leaking amniotic fluid. But she wasn't contracting and her cervix was not dilated. Dr. Olah examined Vanessa and did another sonogram. One of the babies looked fine, but the amniotic sac around "Twin A" was leaking and there was no fluid around the baby at all. It was a serious situation, needing emergency treatment by experts. Dr. Olah arranged to have Vanessa taken by ambulance to the high-risk obstetrics unit at The Johns Hopkins Hospital, seventy-five miles away.

On July 19, Vanessa was admitted to the Hopkins labor and delivery unit. She was diagnosed with ruptured membranes, and put on complete bed rest. By the time she got to Hopkins, contractions had begun. She was only twenty-four weeks pregnant—a full-term pregnancy is thirty-seven to forty weeks. The obstetrician told her that if the babies were born at twenty-four weeks, their survival chances were less than 50 percent. The goal of hospitalization was to allow the babies to stay in her as long as possible. While the technological wonders of neonatal intensive care offer premature infants increasingly improved chances of survival at very young gestational ages, a mother's uterus remains the best place to nurture the unborn infant toward viability.

Vanessa felt tired, hot, frustrated, cranky, and very, very worried.

Rick, when he arrived at Hopkins a few hours later, was also worried, but he felt a sense of security in the fact that Vanessa was being treated at what he had read was the number one hospital in the country. Later, after his surprise encounter with The Divine Healer in the Broadway lobby, he also felt a quiet comfort. *Oh, Lord Jesus, please give our babies life,* he prayed. *Please help us become the happy family we know we can be.*

~

Vanessa was treated with magnesium sulfate, a medication used to stop preterm labor. She also received injections of betamethasone, a steroid that would accelerate the development of the babies' lungs; and intravenous antibiotics. Tests had determined that she was positive for Group B Streptococcus (GBS), a bacterial infection found in the digestive or reproductive tracts of as many as one-third of healthy adult women. GBS usually does not cause problems for the carrier. But when a woman is pregnant, the effects can be calamitous for the baby, causing infections in the bloodstream, respiratory system, and other systems. Premature babies are particularly susceptible.

Vanessa also had a urinary tract infection and later tests turned up *E. coli* bacteria. While she did not feel sick from these infections, her babies could suffer the consequences. Those first couple of days at Hopkins, both Rick and Vanessa were getting bad feelings. *It all seems so negative, there doesn't seem to be much chance,* Rick worried. And the thought *I'm going to lose my babies* went through Vanessa's mind like a refrain.

But the babies' heartbeats were strong, a good sign. Another was the latest sonogram showing the fluid building up again around Twin A. Of course, Vanessa and Rick didn't think of him as "Twin A"–this was Travis, whom the sonograms also showed to be a bit smaller than Troy. She could feel both the babies moving, the fluttery sensations as they floated along the inside of her uterus, the sharper jabs from a knee, an elbow, a foot.

Rick was around most of the time, but he would take breaks from Vanessa's bedside to wander around the hospital, often ending up in the rotunda, where he continued to get unexpected comfort from The Divine Healer. He didn't tell Vanessa about the statue, but he did tell her he was going to pray, which seemed uncharacteristic for him and surprised her. *Gee*, she thought, *all I've ever heard before is him taking God's name in vain.* "Yeah, right," she said when he told her he was going to pray. "You're just going to smoke a cigarette."

As long as Vanessa stayed on the magnesium, there were no contractions, but when the drug was stopped, sharp premature labor pains began again. She was on complete bed rest, with her vital signs checked every four hours. After a few days she started to feel bored and restless. If things continued to go well, she might be able to move around a little and maybe even leave the hospital, the obstetrical resident told her. But one day, after she'd been at the hospital about ten days, as Rick was helping her with her bedpan, he couldn't suppress a gasp. The pan was full of blood. *Oh no*, Vanessa thought, *what next?* She continued bleeding for a few days and there was no more talk of leaving the hospital.

In the middle of the ongoing medical crisis, there was bad news from Cleveland. Vanessa's grandmother, only in her mid-sixties, had been battling cancer for several years and was losing the fight. Vanessa said good-bye to her on the telephone and apologized for having been such an ornery kid. "Grandma, I'm going to have twins," she said, trying to stifle her sobs, and though her grandmother couldn't answer in words, Vanessa had the feeling she understood. Two days later her mother called and told her that her grandmother had died. Don't cry, everyone told Vanessa, it'll just bring more stress to yourself and the babies. She felt that she couldn't grieve the way she wanted to, needed to, and a year later, the unexpressed grief remained a leaden lump within her.

During Vanessa's hospitalization, Rick traveled back and forth to Hagerstown, on leave from his job but keeping appointments with his probation officer. He was home with his parents early in the morning of August 6 when an obstetrical nurse called. "We need you down here," she said. "You're going to be a daddy today. Try to get here by noon." By ten A.M., Rick and his parents were speeding eastward on Route I-70, the now familiar road between Hagerstown and Baltimore, knowing that it was still too early for the babies to have their best shot at a healthy beginning, knowing that something else must have gone wrong.

Awakened by the doctors on their morning rounds, Vanessa felt weak, hot, and achy. "How do you feel?" one of the doctors asked, and she just turned her head and murmured, "Not too good."

"We have a problem," the doctor said. "You've had a high fever all night. That's a sign of infection, that's not good for the babies, and we have to deliver them right away."

Vanessa fell back asleep, barely taking in the news. Someone asked if there was anyone who should be called, and she told them to call Rick at his parents. More antibiotics were added to her IV line, and the magnesium was discontinued. Vanessa started feeling labor pains, and she began to cry. She was wheeled to the delivery room and prepped for an epidural anesthetic. But she was frightened and fighting, calling for Rick, flailing her arms. General anesthesia was administered through her IV. The last thing she remembered was a burning sensation and a fierce wish that Rick was there.

Rick was right outside the door, dressed in scrubs, but kept out of the delivery room because the birth had turned into an emergency procedure. Vanessa was diagnosed with chorioamnionitis—the infection in her body had reached the membranes surrounding the babies. The twins would be delivered by cesarean section—that was much quicker and would reduce the chances of the mother's infection being transmitted to the babies in the birth canal. Once Vanessa was sedated, the attending obstetrician made the incision across her abdomen, rolled back the skin and muscle, then made a second incision through the stretched tissue of her uterus to get the babies out.

The delivery room was filled with more than a dozen doctors and nurses—an obstetrics team for the mother and a neonatal intensive care team for each baby. To an outsider the scene might have looked chaotic, but this was controlled chaos, with a specialized function for every person there. One doctor to deliver the babies, another to listen for the heartbeats, someone else to examine the cord, another to make sure the airway was open. The tension was palpable—at only twenty-seven weeks gestation, everyone knew that special efforts would be necessary for Travis and Troy to have the best chance of surviving and being healthy, and each medical team was prepared for the worst.

Marilee Allen, the attending neonatologist, supervised the care of the babies once they were born. It is a position she has been in many times—she has been a Hopkins neonatologist for more than twenty years—and, as always, she went inward in the last few moments before the babies were delivered, calming herself and preparing for action in what she thought of as her little conversation with God. *God,* she prayed, *please give me the mental strength to be able to focus on what is necessary to bring these babies around, to resuscitate them and keep them alive.*

In the waiting room, Rick broke down in tears, trying to get information from anyone who came out the delivery room door. Two women from the housekeeping staff stayed with him and comforted him. Later, he wondered who these women were who had bolstered his spirits and hopes, but he never found out.

Travis was born first, at 1:32 P.M. His heart rate was below 100 (120 to 170 is normal for a newborn), his breathing labored. His skin was a dusky blue color. Allen quickly placed an oxygen mask over his face, covering both his mouth and nose, and "breathed" for the baby by squeezing a bag attached to the mask. Only after three to four minutes of high-pressure bagging did Travis start moving. Then he was intubated, with a tube through his trachea to his lungs. His Apgar score at one minute was only one. Apgar is the "grading" system for newborns, a quick assessment of heart rate, respiration, color, tone, and reflexes. A healthy responsive baby will receive two points in each category, for a maximum total of ten. Travis got one point for heart rate, and that was all. At five minutes, he got two points for heart rate, but still zeros in the other categories.

In her notes Allen described a "very difficult resuscitation, indicating severe lung disease and sepsis." Once he was intubated, the infant was given the drug Survanta through his breathing tube, a type of treatment called surfactant therapy that improves the function of extremely premature lungs like Travis's.

Rick saw the tiny gurney holding Travis race by, on the way to the neonatal intensive care unit. He had time for only a brief glimpse of his son.

Troy was delivered at 1:34 P.M. He was also blue and floppy, but his breathing was a little bit stronger than his brother's. His heart rate was even lower, however, in the 60s. The intubation was difficult and took three tries. In between the attempts of the respiratory therapist, a doctor was applying chest compression to try to raise the baby's heart rate. After the tube was in, the rate went into the 100s, but Troy's blood pressure was still very low. He had an additional problem—blood was leaking from his umbilical cord, so that was clamped to stop further bleeding. He was put in a plastic bag to reduce heat loss and then he, too, was transported to the NICU.

Rick got a little better introduction to Troy. The doctor stopped and let Rick lift the cover and place a kiss on his baby's tiny head. It would be at least a half hour before all the lines were in the babies and he could visit his sons, the doctor told Rick. Rick headed for the recovery room to see Vanessa. The first thing she remembered as she awakened from the anesthetic was his head coming down toward her, kissing her. "I love you," he whispered. "We have two sons."

Each baby weighed about two pounds six ounces—tiny by any standard but not impossible for survival in this day of neonatology miracles. Still, Travis and Troy presented maximum challenges. In their notes, the neonatologists described both of them as "critically ill." They suffered from immature lungs and probable sepsis—infection in their bloodstream that was circulating throughout their bodies, with the potential to affect all their organs. Premature rupture of membranes and maternal infection put a baby at risk for sepsis. Vanessa had experienced both.

Still woozy from anesthesia, Vanessa wasn't back in her room until early evening and didn't know what danger the babies were in. They were both placed on oscillators—a type of high-frequency ventilator that both inhales and exhales for the patient and is used for babies with the most severely compromised respiratory systems.

Rick and his mother went to see the babies when they were a couple of hours old. He couldn't believe how tiny they were, and how many tubes were running in and out of the small bodies. *So many lines and wires,* he thought, *this is really frightening.* But he was again comforted by the fact that they were getting the best possible treatment. *They're at Johns Hopkins and everything will be okay,* he reassured himself. He was suffused with love as he looked at first Travis, then Troy, both lying still in their Isolettes, their tiny chests rising and falling rapidly from the oscillator. *I thought I loved them as much as I could before they were born,* he marveled, *but God, look at them now. These are my sons!*

Vanessa, coming around, was determined to see the babies too. By about eight-thirty P.M. she felt well enough to make her way from her bed to a wheelchair, and Rick wheeled her the short distance to the NICU. She was only allowed to see Travis for a couple of minutes. He was having difficulties, the NICU staff told her. She held his hand, less than half an inch across, and longed to pick him up. His face looked bruised, the fragile immature skin vulnerable to even a light touch. She felt a flash of anger that she couldn't take him back to her room with her, hold him at her breast, take him home. *It's sure not like on TV, when you get to hold your baby,* she thought resentfully. She kissed his hand, then Rick wheeled her over to see Troy. He looked stronger and more peaceful, and she held his hand and kissed him too. Her anger turned to sorrow and she couldn't keep back the tears as she saw her babies, laid out with tubes snaking in and out of their fragile bodies and machines breathing for them. *Okay,* she said to herself, *you've got to accept this, they told you it would be rough at first.* But another part of her resisted. *This isn't the way it's supposed to be.*

It was time for Rick to share with Vanessa what had given him such peace and solace in the weeks they had been at Hopkins. They took the elevator down to the first floor, and he wheeled her past the Children's Center "zoo," huge stuffed animals in cages. They stopped in the cafeteria and got something to drink, then he wheeled her down the corridor and around the oak staircase into the oldest part of the hospital. Like nearly everyone who first sees the statue, Vanessa was awestruck at its size and presence. Rick showed her the leather-bound books on the pedestals near the statue, where passersby record their thoughts and prayers. Vanessa stood, with difficulty, and wrote her own prayer: *Thank You, God, for giving me my sons. Please keep them okay and help them be able to come home with us.* Then they knelt at the base of the statue, both filled with hope and thanks and fear, and prayed some more. *Thank You, Jesus, for my two sons,* Rick prayed. *Please help everything work out okay for Travis and Troy and all the other babies up there. Please help Vanessa get back to being herself again.*

Back in the room, Vanessa soon fell asleep, exhausted. Rick kissed her and slipped back to the NICU, unable to stay away. He watched Travis and Troy through the glass for a few minutes, then washed his hands and put on a gown so he could touch them. With his big hands he gently touched a tiny finger, an infinitesimal toe, a spot on the head. There were too many tubes to stroke the babies as he wanted to. He stayed for almost an hour. Both the infants seemed to be holding their own. None of the staff told him anything had changed, so he assumed they had stabilized.

He was worn out from the long emotional day and went back to Vanessa's room to try to get some sleep. But almost as soon as Rick left the NICU, Travis's condition worsened. Even with the oscillator, his blood was not getting the oxygen it needed. Raising the settings didn't help. Hand-bagging did help, as it had in the delivery room, but his blood pressure was dropping and a quick blood test showed that he was becoming acidotic. Sodium bicarbonate was given to attempt to reverse a life-threatening pH imbalance, atropine and epinephrine to jolt his slowing heart, and manual chest compressions were begun. But all the advances of modern neonatal technology, and all the fervent prayers of desperately hopeful parents and relatives did not appear to be enough to keep young Travis Allen Canfield Parker alive.

The phone rang in Vanessa's room just after one A.M. It was the NICU, advising her and Rick to get there as soon as they could. Vanessa was so agitated that she couldn't get out of bed, so Rick and the nurse just grabbed the bed and wheeled it down the corridor. At the NICU, someone took hold of the bed and steered it to the left. Vanessa knew that was where Travis was; he must be the baby with the problem. Rick hung back, an unconscious effort to shield himself from bad news. Vanessa saw the crowd around the infant, saw that his lines were out and CPR was being administered. "Stop!" she screamed. "You're hurting my baby!"

It is unlikely that Travis could feel much pain but his heart rate was down to a lethargic thirty-six beats per minute and the chest compressions were not helping him. It was time to stop the efforts to keep him alive. Lee Marban, the attending neonatologist, wrapped him in a blanket and gave him to Vanessa to hold. Tears were streaming down her face. Rick was at her side, also sobbing. The baby took his last breath in his mother's arms. It felt like a quick jarring movement to her, and then nothing. She slumped in despair and handed him to Rick, afraid she would drop him. Marban listened to the tiny chest with a stethoscope and pronounced Travis dead at 1:58 A.M. He had lived just over twelve hours.

Rick looked at the baby in his arms, kissed him, and told him he loved him. Then he and Vanessa dressed him in a soft white cotton sleeper with a little hat and Rick took a picture. He was thinking, *I can't believe this.* He looked at his big competent hands and wondered, *What the hell did I do? What am I being punished for?* There were no answers.

⁓

Vanessa was still fragile from her ordeal. Rick wheeled her back to the room and held her and stroked her and finally got her to go to sleep. There was no sleep for him. Restless and bereft, he found himself again at the Christ statue. He felt he was moving his body around, but his mind was no longer in it. Where was it? He didn't know, maybe off somewhere with poor Travis. Maybe with Troy, holding his own but still critical. He stood and stared at the statue for many minutes, alone in the predawn hours in the rotunda. He turned and grasped the pen at the prayer book and recorded his thoughts, the first of what would be a succession of outpourings in the coming days.

Dear Father,

I don't have contact with You as much as I should but I do believe in You. This morning You received Travis Allen Parker who was only 12 years old. Please let him know that we all miss and love him. We know he'll be okay under Your love. We also ask of You to give us the strength and love to make it through this crisis. We also want You to know that Troy, his twin brother, is fine and he is stabilized. I know that You hear prayers every day but please just let Travis know that we all miss him tremendously. Please

*give [Troy] a chance to become a normal human being. Please
watch over our families as well as the mother Vanessa. Thank
You, God, for Your time.*

> *Forever grateful,*
> *Richard Parker*
> August 7, 1998

Travis's cause of death was listed as "overwhelming sepsis," complicated by hyaline membrane disease, the disease of devastatingly immature lungs. Troy was stabilized, but not really making forward
progress. With an effort, Vanessa and Rick squelched the hovering
presence of fear and dread. They were convinced Troy would survive. The next day both Rick and Vanessa prayed at the foot of The
Divine Healer and recorded their prayers in the book.

Dear Father,

   *Thank You for this day. Thank You for letting us have Troy
for another day. He is still doing the same. Tell Travis that we
miss and love [him] and that his twin brother is still fighting.
Mom and Dad are very grateful to You because You gave us the
chance to see the little guy alive for 12 hours. We are all grateful
to You, Lord Jesus. I would like for You to give us the strength and
courage to hold on. Once again, thank You for everything.*

> *Forever grateful,*
> *Richard Parker*
> August 8, 1998

Vanessa felt a little guilty, a little unworthy. Why should God answer
her prayers? She hadn't exactly been a stalwart believer. But there
was something about the statue and the comfort it offered that made
her feel her prayers would be accepted. She picked up the pen and began without salutation. As the words flowed out of her, she felt she
was talking to God.

Consolation

I don't really know what to say but I love You and need You through this time in my life. I am 21 years old and had beautiful twin boys on the 6th, Troy and Travis. As You know, Travis wasn't strong enough to stay with us and did not share his life with the rest of us, although he was able to last 12 hours. Just let him know that I will always have him with me in my heart and will always pray for him to know his mom. For Troy, he is doing a lot better now and still needs You to be there for him and keep him safe from all the obstacles that come down the road. Just let him be a part of my and Rick's life. Even though he'll always be our baby, just make sure he gets the chance he deserves in life. Even though Travis was taken too soon, take care of my twins and love them like they're Your own. But please give me a chance to take care of Troy as You take care of Travis.

> *Love,*
> *Mommy*
> *Vanessa*
> *AMEN*
> *8-8-98*

She left, but didn't feel she'd said all that was in her heart. A few hours later she returned and wrote more.

Dear God,

I'm just writing down a couple more requests. First I would like You to care for my twin babies and have thoughts about keeping Troy alive and well so I can show You I can be a good mommy. I know I missed my first chance to be a mommy but as You know, no one is perfect. I know that You have good plans for Travis, just let him know that he was loved and always will be. We are going to give him a good rest place and the best respectful service that me and Rick plus family could ever do for him. Just a reminder, I love You and my babies.

> *For Rick's mom and dad, I wish they only knew how much re-*
> *spect I have for them in all they do for and with us. If only they*
> *knew that You gave them the best grandchildren they will always*
> *cherish. Just let them know I love them as if they were my own*
> *parents. I thank You and every one that gives us support and con-*
> *sideration for our feelings. I am having strong thoughts and con-*
> *sideration and utmost respect for You. Just please give me and*
> *Rick the chance to prove our love for You and our babies.*
>
> *Amen,*
> *Vanessa*
> 8-8-98
> *Plus I want to be friends with You and part of Your family too.*

Vanessa recovered quickly from the arduous pregnancy and C-section delivery. She and Rick spent as much time as they could with Troy in the NICU. They were allowed to hold the baby now and then, but not as much as they would have liked. There were some disturbing changes. He was swollen all over—his face, his torso, his limbs. Only one eye seemed to be exempt from the spreading edema. Every time she saw him, Vanessa's tears flowed freely. But she could tell that he could hear her voice and feel her touch. And whenever Rick leaned over him and said, "Hey, this is dad," the infant's unswollen eye opened wide in response.

Vanessa was discharged on August 9. It was difficult to leave Troy, but they had to get to Hagerstown and make the necessary preparations to bury Travis. Rick and Vanessa left the hospital in the evening, after a visit to The Divine Healer. Once again, they both wrote in the book.

> *Dear Father,*
> *Thank You for giving us Troy Allen Canfield for 1 more day.*
> *We are truly grateful. Please watch over him as we bury his*

brother and keep him warm and safe. Please give all the doctors
the strength and courage to do for him. Watch over and guide
Vanessa and I as we leave for a couple of days and do this. Watch
over everybody here that's sick and love and keep them at peace.
Tell Travis that we love and miss him and we know You'll take
good care of him. Watch over Vanessa and I please.

> *Truly grateful,*
> *Richard Parker*
> *8-9-98*

Dear God,
   Take best care of Troy since we are not going to be here. Be-
cause we'll be taking care of his brother twin Travis. Please let
him be the best he can be.

> *Amen,*
> *Mommy*
> *Vanessa*
> *8-9-98*

It was tough being home with no babies. This wasn't the way Rick
and Vanessa had envisioned parenthood—making funeral arrangements, calling the cemetery, the florist, friends and relatives. They
also called the Hopkins NICU several times a day to get updates on
Troy, and he continued to hang on without really improving. Sometimes Vanessa would just sit and cry, and it broke Rick's heart to see
her. He proposed that they help run the bingo game at the carnival
that was in town, and it did give them something to do.

   At the NICU, Troy faced increasing complications. At the age of
one week, he was receiving a flood of medications—antibiotics to
counter the infections, dopamine to raise his blood pressure, transfu-
sions to treat low platelets and white cells in his blood, dobutamine to

strengthen his heartbeat, insulin to regulate elevated glucose. His lung collapsed and a tube was inserted in his chest to reinflate it. In the middle of the week, Rick and Vanessa went to Hopkins for a visit and heard still more bad news. Christopher Golden, a neonatology fellow, explained that Troy had developed significant bleeding in his head, in both hemispheres of his brain. Bleeding was graded on a scale of one to four, with four the worst. Troy was four-plus on both sides, Golden told them gently. Here was something new to consider: if he did survive there was now a "high likelihood" that he would be disabled, either cognitively, or in his motor skills, or by blindness, or deafness, or a combination.

"Despite this grim prognosis," Golden wrote in Troy's progress notes, "the parents do not want to withdraw support at this point."

To Vanessa, all these dire possibilities didn't matter. It was just something they would have to deal with. This was still her baby, and she wouldn't love him any less if he were disabled. But she couldn't keep herself from wondering. *Is someone out to get me? People do worse things than I've done in my life and they don't get punished like this.*

Rick was glad the doctor was being honest. But he heard the words thinking, *I'm not losing faith,* as if he was trying to convince himself. He had a picture in his mind of losing Travis and he thought, *It's impossible for us to go through this twice, something good has to come out of this.*

Another thought also crept in. *If we lose Troy too, I'll never be able to pray again.*

Marilee Allen's progress notes the next day emphasized the gulf between Troy's condition and his parent's expectations. "This child remains critically ill," she wrote. His parents "understand the severity of his illness, but have a strong belief that he will survive." She went on to catalog a list of pessimistic markers: his urine output was down, his blood pressure was down, his blood glucose was up and down, his hematocrit was down, he was very swollen and his skin was discolored, he had virtually no spontaneous movement. "I am concerned about perfusion [blood flow] to major organs because of his overwhelming sepsis," she added. "His gut and kidney have been affected."

~

Travis was buried Saturday morning, August 15, nine days after he was born. He was laid to rest in Hagerstown's Rose Hill Cemetery, which has a section set apart for very young children. A weeping willow and two ceramic cherubs frame the site. About twenty-five people were at the funeral at Minnich Funeral Home, conducted by pastor Robert Fitz, a friend of Rick's dad, from the Bible Church in nearby Waynesboro, Pennsylvania. At the small memorial service at the cemetery, Vanessa and Rick hung on to each other for comfort, feeling numb and drained. They put toys in Travis's tiny coffin—a little stuffed Tweety Bird, a teddy bear rattle, a ceramic figurine of a cat in a moon. A picture of Travis Tritt looked down from the propped-open lid of the coffin during the service and also accompanied baby Travis on his final journey.

During the service, the pastor asked the question in everyone's mind: "Why would a loving God give to Travis the precious gift of life, and then take it away after twelve short hours in this world?" But he was as empty of answers as anyone. "Even if we could explain why Travis left his family, the explanation wouldn't begin to heal your broken hearts," he told the gathered mourners. "We don't need reasons today; we need spiritual help to accept the sorrow and be able to go back to life better able to carry the burdens."

Pastor Fitz prayed for strength and comfort for the bereaved parents:

When King David's little son died, David said, "I shall go to him, but he shall not return to me" (2 Samuel 12:23). Where was David going? He tells us in Psalm 23: "I will dwell in the house

*of the Lord forever." David knew he would one day go to heaven
and there meet his son.*

*What a blessing and comfort to know where your loved ones are
and that you can meet them again. . . . The Bible says, "Jesus
took them in His arms and blessed them." Let Him take you in
His strong arms today and bless you. He can and will do it, if you
welcome Him into your life.*

That evening, Rick and Vanessa decided to work the carnival for a
few hours to get their minds off their loss. But Vanessa was nervous
and kept having a feeling that someone was trying to get in touch.
They left work early and at home saw on the caller ID that the NICU
had called. When they phoned back, the nurse said Troy had taken a
turn for the worse. They should get to Hopkins as soon as possible.

Vanessa fainted, and when she came to, started throwing up and
hyperventilating. Rick made a bunch of fast phone calls—his parents, Vanessa's mom and brother. Everyone converged at Rick's parents' home and they piled into three cars to make the trip to
Baltimore. When they got to the NICU, the nurse said sadly, "He's
still here. I guess he wanted to hold on for you."

Frances Northington was the attending neonatologist. For two
days Troy had experienced progressive respiratory failure and responded only briefly to adjustments in his lung support. His blood
pressure and oxygen blood level were getting lower and lower. By the
time Vanessa and Rick and the rest of the family got to the NICU, he
was not responding to the maximum support possible and was deteriorating rapidly. "There's not even a millionth of a chance anymore," the doctor told the family. "We just laid one to rest," Rick
cried. "There's got to be some chance. Some good has to come out of
this."

The doctor asked Vanessa and Rick if they were ready to order
discontinuation of the life supports. They couldn't do it. Vanessa was
weeping and screaming, "No, no, this can't happen." Rick felt rage

Consolation

suffuse him. *What kind of God would do this?* He left the room and went running down the hall. Vanessa gave him a couple of minutes, and then went after him. She knew where he had fled.

As she entered the rotunda, Rick walked out of the shadows at the foot of The Divine Healer, and put his arms around Vanessa. "I don't feel that warm feeling that I usually do when I'm here," he said desolately.

"Hon, we have to do this, you see that Troy's suffering," Vanessa murmured. "We've done all we can do and now we have to let him go and we have to do it together." They hugged. "I don't want to let go but I don't want to see him suffer anymore," she whispered. Rick felt his anger at God drain from his body, but there was nothing positive to replace it, only harsh grief, so strong he could feel it physically. Vanessa wanted to comfort him but felt such an emptiness in herself that there was no place from where she could summon comfort. *A God who could let this happen couldn't care very much about me,* she thought bleakly.

They went back to the NICU, watched while the tubes in Troy and the breathing machine were removed. Everyone got a chance to hold him. Then Rick sat in a rocking chair with him. "It's daddy time," he whispered. He held the infant until his little heart stopped beating. Northington confirmed the death at 3:22 A.M. Before they left the hospital, Rick found himself again at the statue. In the book, he poured out his anguish and bewilderment.

Dear God,

Why do You make us feel this way? Why did You take our sons from us? We did nothing to deserve this pain and suffering. We buried Travis today only to take his brother's life this evening? Why did You do this?

[Rick]
8-16-98

Young Souls

A year has passed. On a hot August afternoon, Rick and Vanessa stop at the Rose Hill Cemetery to visit Travis's and Troy's graves. The weeping willow is in full foliage, lush and green. The two small headstones are in a row of about a dozen, most of the dates indicating lifespans of less than a year. The twins' names and dates are engraved on their headstones. Each stone also says "Beloved son of Richard and Vanessa" and has a little heart engraved on it. A white and blue Styrofoam cross is mounted at each grave. Rick and Vanessa, her mom and brother, his parents, other friends often stop by with flowers. The twins have certainly not been forgotten.

Vanessa and Rick stand at the graves, silent. There are no other people around, and the sounds of the outside world are muffled by the trees surrounding the cemetery. Mommy and Daddy are sharing a private moment with their twin boys. After a few minutes they bend down and kiss the gravestones. They walk off, arm in arm, and Rick bends from his six and a half feet to hug her. They are both teary-eyed.

Vanessa is pregnant. Due at the end of October, she is already beyond the time when Travis and Troy were born, and this pregnancy is going smoothly. Once again, she is carrying twins—this time a boy and a girl. She didn't take fertility pills either time to cause a multiple pregnancy. She smiles serenely when asked about this propensity to carry twins, and points upwards. "It's Him," she says quietly. "I don't have any doubts anymore."

Her faith has grown enormously in the year since Travis and Troy died. Rick's faith, she believes, pulled her in. Not that it was easy or straightforward. In those first weeks after the babies died, she felt she was floundering and alone, that the world was an impossible place. She and Rick even separated for a while, but that only lasted ten days. When she found out she was carrying twins again, she cried her eyes out. "He's watching over us," Rick says with calm certainty. "He's going to make sure things are okay this time. I believe everything is done for a reason. I don't know the reason and probably never will."

Consolation

~

Postscript: Hailey and Cameron Canfield Parker were born at Washington County Hospital on October 16, 1999, about the due date of Travis and Troy a year earlier. These babies weighed nearly seven pounds each, more than twice the weight of their ill-fated brothers. The pregnancy was fairly uneventful, although Vanessa was huge at the end, carrying what amounted to a nearly fourteen-pound baby. Vanessa and Rick thank God for their healthy babies, and the second chance that can come in the wake of tragedy.

> *Jesus loves children, Jesus loves me,*
> *Jesus loves you, with love tenderly.*
> *Jesus loves all, no matter how small,*
> *That's why we love Jesus,*
> *Better than all.*

—CHILDREN'S SONG READ AT TROY'S FUNERAL

EMANUEL "NICK" GERONDIS
A Mother's Fear

Lord, where is my son? Lord, please send him home to me now, let him just walk through that door. Dear Lord, please let him be all right.

Where was Nick? Donna Kaye Reed came in from walking the dog, an hour-long walk in the park, and her twelve-year-old son had gone out. She couldn't find him. It was late, getting to midnight on a September Sunday in 1999, and no sign of the boy. She didn't trust the neighborhood—she knew there was drug dealing going on just a few blocks away. She was apprehensive about the boys Nick had been running with—most were older than he, they drank and perhaps used drugs. Weapons too she feared. Anxiety clutched at her and wouldn't let go. Where was Nick?

He'd kissed her good-bye before she went out. "I love you," he said, and she grinned at his quick, spontaneous affection.

"You love me? What do you want?" Donna joked.

"No, I don't want anything."

"Come walk the dog with me."

"I don't want to tonight, maybe tomorrow I will."

He had been like this since he was a little boy. "I love you, Nicky," Donna would tell him, and from the time he could talk he'd fling open his arms and respond, "I love you more." She was glad he still said it, although these days he was chafing at restrictions, wanting to be a grown-up and not having to report to her all the time. This night, as she was going out, she shot back an admonition:

"Don't go to Ash Street."

"Don't worry, Mom, I won't."

Now he was gone, and she didn't know where. For the past three weeks, Donna and Nick had been staying with her mother in Woodberry, a neighborhood on the southern edge of The Johns Hopkins University campus, near the Jones Falls and light-rail tracks. It was only temporary—she had lost the house she rented in Glen Burnie, a suburb south of Baltimore, when a relative of the landlord unexpectedly moved to the area. She planned to move back, out of the city, as soon as she could find a place. Woodberry was once a safe area, working-class people who mostly owned their homes and contributed to the community. But in recent years, the neighborhood had gone downhill. Earlier that summer, a fourteen-year-old boy who lived on their street and was friends with Nick had been stabbed to death during a robbery. Ash Street, in particular, a couple blocks away, was known as an illegal drug market, especially for crack cocaine.

"Nicky!" Donna yelled as she came into the house, but the only answer was from her mother, in the back room. "Don't come in, go look for your son," Karen Reed called. She'd heard him leave while she was in the bathtub, but he hadn't told her where he was going. As Donna started knocking on doors where some of Nick's friends lived, she couldn't stop thinking about the boy who had been murdered.

No one had seen Nick. "If you see my son, tell him I want him home," she told people. An awful feeling was building, an ominous premonition that something was terribly wrong. *Please, God, be with him, send him home to me. Please, Jesus, let him be okay.* She ran home and dialed 311, the nonemergency police number. It was almost one A.M., and she was trying to explain exactly where she lived to the operator, becoming exasperated as she couldn't make herself understood, when she saw two women get out of a car and walk toward her door. She knew them—they lived on Ash Street and were both named Lisa. She dropped the phone and stepped outside.

"Nick's been shot in the head," blurted one of the Lisas. "His brains were splattered all over the street. You'd better come quick."

Donna screamed and fell to the ground. She rose and went into the house. "Mom, they're telling me he's dead," she said. She picked up the phone again and this time called 911. "Was there a shooting on Ash Street tonight?" she asked the emergency operator. She was shrieking. "Calm down," the operator told her. "They're en route to Sinai Hospital. The best way for you to find out what's going on would be to talk to the police officers at the scene."

A neighbor drove Donna the short distance to Ash Street, and when she saw the flashing lights and cordoned area, she knew her worst fears were being realized. "It's my son, my son who was shot," she yelled at the police officer who tried to keep her from the scene. Finally someone told her he was on his way to the hospital—Sinai, a couple of miles away. And he wasn't dead, he'd had a pulse when he was taken from the scene. Shaking and crying, Donna found someone to drive her to the hospital. The police wanted her to stay and answer some questions, but she had to get to Nick.

When she finally saw him, in the emergency room treatment cubicle, she couldn't believe how bad he looked. If she hadn't known who he was, she wouldn't have recognized her own son. His head was swollen to half again its normal size. He was unconscious, unmoving, breathing through a tube down his throat attached to a ventilator. The entrance wound on the left side of his head was covered with a gauze bandage. "No-o-o-o-o!" Donna howled, and her knees buckled; she slid down the wall to the floor and sat there sobbing, her head on her knees. Her mom had met her at the hospital, and she helped Donna get up. Donna knew she had to keep it together for Nick, had to make sure he got the best possible treatment. She leaned over him and told him the biggest lie she'd ever told. "You look great," she said. "Everything is going to be okay."

In the emergency room, Nick was given Dilantin, an antiseizure drug; mannitol to control the brain swelling; an antibiotic to prevent infection, and a tetanus shot. A decision was quickly made to transfer to him to The Johns Hopkins Hospital, the regional center for pediatric trauma cases. Donna rode the seven miles in the ambulance with her son. Her faith in God and Jesus had come to her rescue during hard times in the past, and now, as the ambulance sped down the Jones Falls Expressway and across the city, lights flashing, she tried to calm herself with prayer, to ward off the one thought she couldn't keep from surfacing: *Please, God, don't let him die. Don't let him die. Don't let him die. Don't let him die.*

⁓

Donna Kaye Reed grew up in Baltimore and San Diego. Her parents separated when she was four, divorced when she was eight. She hardly saw her father at all, and her relationship with her mother could be abrasive and volatile. Mother and daughter were both high-strung and contentious, and arguments could get ugly, especially as Donna moved through her teen years.

When Donna was seven, her grandfather gave her a Bible. Whenever she could, she went to her mother's Methodist church and enjoyed the experience—her life could be uncertain sometimes, but she felt comfortable in church, a sense of belonging that she didn't have much of elsewhere. God and Jesus loved her, she heard in church and read in the Bible, and that was a reassuring thought because she often felt there wasn't much love in her life. *Even when you don't have love anywhere else,* she thought, *God loves us all.*

About the time her grandfather gave her a Bible, she first saw the Christ statue under the dome at Hopkins. She was there with her mother to visit a friend, and they came in through the Broadway entrance. *Wow, this is so huge, so beautiful,* young Donna thought as she came up the short flight of steps and into the rotunda and confronted The Divine Healer. His outreaching arms seemed warmly embracing and, young as she was, she felt the peace that so many describe around the statue. She moved closer and saw the wounds of crucifixion in His hands and feet, and that brought tears to her eyes. *God is here,* she thought. *There's no doubt about that.*

In the years that followed she didn't forget God, but sometimes the idea of Him seemed more remote than when she was a girl. She made some bad choices. She became pregnant when she was in the eleventh grade and quit school. Danielle was born in 1979 when Donna was seventeen. Donna loved her baby, but being a mother was hard work and the baby's father didn't want to have anything to do with either of them. She never got a penny of child support from him and soon lost contact. Danielle was a difficult child, emotional and high-strung like her mother and grandmother, and family life was often tumultuous.

Donna wanted to move beyond minimum wage jobs and started computer school in 1979, earning her high school equivalency the next year. She had a variety of jobs—retail, waitressing, clerical, receptionist. She had some boyfriends but no relationships that amounted to much. She stayed in the Baltimore area and was living with her mom in 1984 when she met Nicolaos Gerondis one night at a bar. He was from Greece and had come to the United States for employment opportunity more than fifteen years earlier. He had a high-paying but dangerous job, sandblasting and painting steel bridges. Donna was smitten the first time she saw him. She found out he was married but separated, and after a few months he convinced her he was serious about ending his marriage. They never lived together—Nick called himself a "free bird" and was wary of getting tied down—but spent much of their time with each other and Donna was delighted when she became pregnant in early 1986.

Emanuel Nicolaos Gerondis, called Nicky, was born in Baltimore County on October 6, 1986. Nick, his dad, was intimidated at first by the prospect of a baby. He had broken his arm in a fall from a bridge a month before the baby was born and had to take off work for nearly a year. This provided plenty of opportunity for him to get to know his infant son, and he quickly learned how much fun a kid can be. He left the United States when his son was five, deported because of criminal activities, and then contact was limited to frequent letters and phone calls and a month-long visit to Greece when Nicky was eleven.

Young Nicky was a sweet, generous, affectionate boy. Donna

took him and Danielle to church and beamed as her friends told her what a joy he was. They moved around a bit, and as he got older, he knew how much she wished she could buy a house and have a place where they could stay put. "Mom, when I grow up, I'm going to buy two houses, one for you and one for me," he promised her. He loved animals and didn't understand harsh people. As he approached his teens, he started playing football in pickup games in his neighborhood. He also loved video games and spent hours fooling around on a computer at the public library. He was big for his age, with a chubby face and short brown hair. He looked older than his years, and most of the Woodberry kids thought he was at least sixteen.

Nick had some problems too. When he was seven, he was diagnosed with attention deficit disorder, ADD. He took Ritalin, which helps children with this disorder focus on tasks and curb inappropriate impulses. To Donna, it didn't seem he was all that hyperactive, which is often a feature of the disorder, but she saw through the years that his school performance depended on whether he had a teacher who took a special interest and made an effort to get through to him. Donna volunteered in his classrooms so she could see for herself what the atmosphere was and how Nick was handling it.

It was soon clear that Nick couldn't learn with the distractions of a regular classroom, and he was placed in special schools. He did well in middle school at the Children's Guild, a school that specializes in learning disordered or emotionally disturbed youngsters. He had just started the eighth grade when Donna lost their place and they moved in with her mom in Baltimore. At the time of the shooting, she was trying to figure out how she was going to get Nick back and forth to school until they could move. She was working, shuttling cars for a car rental company, but didn't have a vehicle of her own.

As pieced together later from eyewitness accounts, newspaper reports, and the police investigation, Nick Gerondis was shot in the head during a robbery attempt around one A.M., Monday, September 20, 1999. Just seconds before, the shooter had held his gun to the head of a sixteen-year-old boy in the group who handed over fifty dollars. The robber then turned to Nick, who was sitting in a porch chair on the sidewalk. When Nick said he had no money, the man shot him. Nick's chin dropped to his chest, his blood quickly drenching his clothing. Most of the other kids scattered. Someone called 911 to report the shooting, but Nick sat bleeding for precious minutes before emergency medical help arrived.

Traumatic brain injuries (TBI) kill fifty thousand Americans a year, and the highest risk is among adolescent boys. About eighty thousand TBI victims are discharged from hospitals each year with permanent disabilities. Most head injuries are from auto accidents, violence, or falls. As stricter enforcement and growing public awareness have increased the use of seat belts, resulting in fewer head injuries from car crashes, firearms have passed motor vehicles as the largest single cause of TBI mortality in the United States. Brain injuries caused by violence are by far the most lethal—91 percent of firearm-related head injuries end in death.

Donna didn't know these statistics when Nick was taken to Hopkins, but the knowledge that her son's odds of survival were less than 10 percent wouldn't have affected her thinking much. Wrapped around the images of those dawn hours—the frantic ambulance ride, the dread she felt in the Hopkins emergency room, the doctors who shook their heads when they talked to her—were her prayers: *Please, God, I know You love him more than I do, but let him stay with me. Let my son stay with me.* From the start, none of the medical personnel had anything good to tell her about Nick, and Donna felt like she was falling to pieces. It was all she could do to keep from screaming in anguish, and sometimes she did scream.

Nick arrived at Hopkins at 4:56 A.M. and his neurological assessment found no motor response, no verbal response, no eye opening, no pupil response, no corneal reflexes, and no sensory responses in his arms and legs. Comas range from light to heavy, depending on the extent of the victim's responses, and are graded on a measure called the Glasgow Coma Scale. Points are given in each of three areas: eye response, verbal response, and motor response, with a total maximum of fifteen. Less than eight points is classified as a severe head injury. Nick scored a three—the lowest possible score, the deepest level of coma.

Within minutes, Nick's spine was X rayed and he was found to have no spinal injury. His heartbeat was irregular. The CAT scan of his head showed extensive bleeding in his brain from a bullet that had entered in the left side, through the parietal lobe, which is involved with sensation, language and mathematical ability, long-term memory, and voluntary motion. The bullet, which damaged both halves of Nick's brain, broke into fragments in his head, and the fragments remained. Because the damage was so widespread, surgery was not a treatment option. At 5:09 A.M., he was moved to the pediatric intensive care unit (PICU), the destination of almost all pediatric trauma patients.

Nick's brain was swelling dangerously. In the closed cavity of the skull, there is little room for the brain to swell without causing serious impairment or death. An intracranial monitor kept track of the pressure within Nick's head. Like blood pressure, intracranial pressure (ICP) is measured in amount of pressure needed to raise a column of mercury (Hg) one millimeter. Normal ICP is 0 to 10 mmHg. Nick's was about 45 when he came in, with counts in the 60s and 80s and spikes above 100 in the next days. He was put on a high dose of a barbiturate, which reduces swelling by decreasing metabolic rate and blood volume and constricting the blood vessels in the brain.

"It's not good," Joanne Natale, the PICU fellow who treated Nick the first day, told Donna and Karen. "You'd better think about saying your good-byes and get anyone who loves him here with you. Nick's injury is critical and his survival is unlikely." In her progress note, she outlined the life supports in place for Nick, but concluded, "the outlook for neurological recovery is poor. The mother understands Nick is likely to die despite these efforts."

Donna said she understood, but she refused to believe it. She was told to move away from Nick's bedside as the PICU team worked on him to stabilize his breathing, heart rate, fluid intake, and medications. She found a phone and called the American embassy in Athens, gave the people she talked to all the information she had about Nick's father, and asked them to locate him because his son was critically ill and in a coma. The Baltimore Police Department also went to work to help get Nick, Sr., to his son's bedside.

The next day Donna prayed with Charles Thomas, the on-call chaplain, and in his notes he wrote that she was appreciative of the time he spent with her. She asked him to suggest Bible readings that would comfort her in this crisis, and he recommended Psalms 100–103 and the fifth chapter of James. Thomas concluded, "James 5:14 is appropriate for her. Her story is much pain, losses, and changes. She feels she was guilty of doing some wrong, and her sins were visited upon her son. She said she believes God is with him and will take care of him."

> *Is any sick among you? Let him call for the elders of the church; and let them pray over him, anointing him with oil in the name of the Lord. And the prayer of faith shall save the sick, and the Lord shall raise him up; and if he have committed sins, they shall be forgiven him.*
>
> —JAMES 5:14–15

Donna spent the next days at Nick's bedside, talking to him, rubbing his arm and hand, stroking his leg, praying to see a response, but there was none. She kept her eyes fixed on the monitors, looking for a change that signaled improvement. But the read-outs on the machines that kept Nick alive offered little hope. He remained on maximum life support. A CAT scan on Tuesday, his second day, showed that some parts of his brain were not receiving blood flow, and the swelling remained pervasive.

Kathleen Corbett, an Episcopal priest and onetime nurse, was the Hopkins chaplain on duty in the PICU when Nick was there. She had only been on the Hopkins chaplaincy staff a week, and this case would be a consuming one for her. She saw Nick two days after he was shot, and after the nurses explained his condition, she went to his bedside, held his hand, and prayed for him. *Lord, shed Your grace on this boy, and on his family. Please give the doctors and nurses the understanding they need. Please comfort this boy and be with him during whatever will happen to him. Amen.*

Kathy went downstairs to her office and was confronted by a woman she didn't know. "Does God punish people for being evil?" asked the woman, who was tearful and desperate looking. "Did I do something to deserve this? Did my son do something to deserve this?"

As she attempted to comfort the woman, Kathy realized she was talking to the mother of the boy she had just prayed for. Donna was agitated, confused, and very frightened—afraid of what had happened to Nick and what he was going through, afraid of what it meant for her. Over the next six weeks, Kathy prayed with Donna and comforted her nearly every day.

Donna was praying for a miracle. "Johns Hopkins is a place of miracles," she told Kathy. "I know they can perform a miracle on Nicky." Kathy was aware of Nick's condition and his pessimistic prognosis and thought Donna was unrealistic to cling to hope of recovery. But she supported her prayers. "Do you think I'm wrong?" Donna asked her after a discouraging meeting with Nick's doctors. "Wrong for what?" Kathy asked. "Wrong for praying for a miracle and not giving up hope? That's your job, you're his mom, you cling to your hope."

They talked, too, about Donna's anger. At times Donna would scream at God, "How could You let this happen? How could You let me live my life with so much trouble to come to this?" Kathy soothed her. "Don't give up on God," the chaplain consoled. "It's all right to be mad at God, because God knows your heart."

In meetings with the doctors, Donna sometimes walked out in tears when the news was too hard for her to bear. Or she looked out the window and didn't listen, or put her head down on the table with her hands over her ears. Nick stabilized somewhat, but there were no signs of recovery—he still needed maximum supports to stay alive and received them, at Donna's insistence. Coping became a little easier for Donna when Nick's father arrived from Europe ten days after the shooting. They got along well, unlike Donna and her mother. Despite their shared concern for Nick, Donna and Karen couldn't agree on much and got into emotional shouting matches at the hospital, to the horror of the PICU staff.

For the first two weeks Nick was in the hospital, Donna barely left his bedside. After a few days, though, she remembered the Christ statue that had had such an impact on her when she was a girl. It wasn't difficult to find her way to the figure under the dome, and she was struck again by the power of the sculpture. She prayed: *Please, God, hear my prayers. Please let my son live, please let him come back to a semblance of what he was before he was shot. If we can't have him exactly the way he was before, that's okay. Please, God, thank You for the wonderful son You let me have, and please understand my selfishness in wanting to keep him.*

After a few visits to the statue, she realized that people wrote prayers in the books on the nearby pedestals, and added her own:

Dear God,

Thank You for my wonderful son. I want to also thank You for every day that You have allowed him to stay with me. I thank You also that his heart is still strong after they have taken him off the blood pressure medicine. I pray every day that it is in Your will to heal him and to heal all. Let him stay with all of us that love him. Is it selfish to want to keep him with me a little longer? I know if

Consolation

he has to go with You , he will be in a better place. Please forgive me for wanting him to stay with me.

Your daughter,
Donna K. R.
10-3-99

Days and then weeks went by, and Nick Gerondis clung to life. His ankles were splinted to keep them from contracting, as happens with the joints of coma patients. He was treated for sores on his heels, often a problem for people who are bedridden. The longer he stayed alive, the less chance there was of sudden death. But there was also less chance for recovery—most likely, the gunshot had caused irreparable brain damage. The neurological formula states that the longer the period before recovery from coma begins, the more limited the recovery. Donna felt numb as she sat by her son's bed, stroked him, and talked to him. She seized upon anything as a sign of improvement—when the doctors decided Nick no longer needed medications to keep his blood pressure at an adequate level, hope crept in. But there was no discernible improvement.

On October 5, David Nichols, director of the PICU and attending physician for the month, described Nick as "sedated, unresponsive to verbal stimuli, withdraws from painful stimuli, occasional cough." It was decided to wean him from the high dose of barbiturate, to see if with the lifting of the barbiturate coma, the trauma coma might also lift. Again, no change was noted.

On the following day, Nick's thirteenth birthday, Donna got him a cake and birthday balloons, but she couldn't light the candles on the cake because of the oxygen in the room. On the same day, pediatric neurologist Rebecca Ichord did an extensive neurological workup of Nick. She described "minimal signs of neurologic function": some reflexive withdrawal from pain in his legs; some breathing "over the ventilator," which meant he was taking breaths on his own; and occasional sluggish reaction of his pupils to light. But there was no other response to light or sound and no voluntary movement. His intracranial pressure remained elevated, spiking sometimes to 100. "My assessment is that this young man has suffered irreversible bihemispheral and brainstem injury . . . and has a very high probability of remaining in a vegetative state if he survives," Ichord noted. She suggested, and the PICU resident agreed, that the family should be offered the option of withdrawing life supports and letting Nick die.

Donna wouldn't consider it. She exploded at the doctors. "I don't want to hear this," she screamed. "Don't even think about pulling the plug!" She became increasingly agitated and the doctors suggested that she could benefit from a psychiatric consultation. She knew that she needed help and support, and was willing to accept it from any quarter, but when she visited the psychiatric outpatient clinic, she was told she would have to wait hours to be seen, and she didn't want to wait.

Back at Nick's bedside, Kathy Corbett was visiting, and she put her arm around Donna and prayed for her and her son. *Please, God,* the chaplain prayed, *spare Nick from any pain and suffering. Allow the physicians and nurses to understand his healing process and give him comfort. Give patience to Donna and Karen, and allow them to understand what You have in mind for Nick.* Later that week, Donna prayed at the foot of The Divine Healer, and found some solace, although her heart still ached and all her choices seemed unacceptable. Discontinue life supports? Impossible. Stay like this? Almost as difficult. All she could pray for was peace for her son. She wrote in the book:

> *Dear Jesus,*
> *Please allow Emanuel to have memories of beautiful things while in this coma state, and please I beseech You to allow Your heart to let him heal.*
> *O Heavenly Father, thank You.*
>
> 10-9-99

Consolation

The words the doctors used in their notes about Nick are part of medical jargon, but harshly descriptive and hopeless sounding to the layperson: he was in a "vegetative" state; he was "neurologically devastated." Donna couldn't bear to hear the words and refused to make management decisions beyond continuing full life supports. "I can't deal with this, I'm not ready for this," she told the doctors. She was heartened by indications that Nick's breathing initiative was improving and wrote at the statue:

> *Dear Lord,*
>
> *Lord Jesus, thank You for letting my son breathe again. I am praising You now and always. I still pray for You to help guide me in his rehabilitation. Again, thank You for this wondrous miracle. Help aid in the rest of his recovery.*
>
> Donna
> 10-14-99

Nick was still far from breathing on his own, however, and on October 15 he underwent two surgical procedures—one to place a permanent breathing tube in his throat to replace the intubation tube that ran down his throat from his mouth; the other to place a feeding tube in his stomach to replace feeding through his nose. He tolerated both procedures well and was transferred back to the PICU in stable condition. Six days later he was judged stable enough to be moved to the pediatric intermediate care unit, but the transfer summary of his condition was no more encouraging than previous reports. "He is completely debilitated with a very poor chance of any recovery; no higher brain function and . . . no expectation of improvement," his chart read. Two days later, his Glasgow Coma Score was assessed at 3 to 4.

At her son's bedside, Donna peppered the doctors and nurses with questions. How can you be sure his function won't recover? Why can't he learn things all over again, like a baby? How can you rule out a miracle? In cases like Nick's, doctors are usually reluctant to speak in absolutes, and everyone acknowledged that the unexpected can and sometimes does happen in coma cases. But Nick, no longer sedated on barbiturates, showed no signs of spontaneous recovery. When Ichord examined him on October 27, three weeks after her initial evaluation, she found "no eye opening, purposeful movement, or response to voice or visual stimuli; no response to sound, light or touch; persistent coma." She added, "prognosis for recovery to normal is nil, most likely will remain in vegetative state . . . [but] . . . mother rejected any further discussion of care strategies which limit life support measures."

Because Nick was medically stable, it was time to look for other placement—an acute care hospital like Hopkins was no longer appropriate. He was accepted at the Mount Washington Pediatric Hospital, a children's rehabilitation facility in north Baltimore, and would be transferred as soon as a bed became available. While Nick's first weeks in the hospital were covered by Donna's health insurance, she left her job to spend all her time with him, and subsequent costs were covered by the state's medical assistance program.

As these arrangements were made through late October, Donna was positive she saw new responses from Nick. She spent more time than the doctors with her son; she couldn't expect them to see what she saw. The first sign was a frown on his face, and little mouth movements. She was sure this wasn't the reflexive-type movement that the doctors had told her was a result of brainstem activity and not conscious or purposeful. Then she saw him move his foot, in response to her. "C'mon, Nicky, you move that foot, let's see what you can do," she pleaded with him one afternoon. She was always begging him to move, to communicate, to acknowledge her in some way, and this time she was sure he did. Donna shared her joy with Kathy Corbett and poured out her thanks to The Divine Healer.

Dear Lord,

Thank You for all of Your miracles . . . Especially for the miracle of Emanuel, thank You for all of my time with him. Thank

Consolation

*You for not allowing that bullet to bring him to You. . . . Thank
You for the miracle You have given my son.*
                                        Donna Reed
                                        10-28-99

~~~~~

On November 5, forty-seven days after he was shot, Nick Gerondis
was transferred to Mount Washington. His discharge summary described his condition as "poor." Donna rode in the ambulance with
him, back up the Jones Falls Expressway, almost retracing the ambulance route from the first hospital where he was treated. Donna felt
good about moving on, especially after the battles she'd had with so
many doctors at Hopkins. As they made the short drive, she thought
about the affirmative power of love, as she had read in the Bible. *Love
does no wrong to anyone, so love satisfies all of God's requirements* [Ro-
mans 13:10]. She believed that the strength of her love, the force of
her will, and the power of her prayers could bring Nicky back to her.

Miracles are often thought of as sudden and dramatic occur-
rences, but Donna Reed was positive she saw miracles daily in the
tiny incremental advances her son started making in the sixth and
seventh weeks following his shooting. Every day she saw him do
something different. It was like seeing a baby develop—although the
progress wasn't as straightforward or predictable.

Rehabilitation is a lengthy process—Mount Washington is a
long-term facility, and Nick's stay there would be measured in
months, not days or weeks. In children, the brain has a tremendous
capacity for healing. Ajoke Ajayi-Akintade, a developmental pediatrician who was Nick's primary doctor at Mount Washington, has
seen and read of enough cases of brain-injured children to know that
extent of recovery cannot be predicted. In the rehab hospital, Nick
was put in a special chair so he could sit up. He received respiratory
therapy, thumping on his chest to keep his lungs clear; and physical
therapy to keep supple the contracted muscles in his arms and legs,
hands, and feet. He had an hour a day of "school," where he was pre-

sented with simple information and his teacher tried to get responses from him.

Gradually, the responses came. After five months, there was no doubt that Nick was conscious and able to communicate. He smiled, he laughed, he turned his head toward sound. He shook or nodded his head in response to questions. He could see, although probably not much from his left eye. He recognized people from their voices and was clearly delighted when his mother came into the room. "Nicky, are you a girl?" Donna asked him playfully, and he vehemently shook his head in a negative response. "Are you my boy?" she asked, and he nodded affirmatively.

By mid-April, as Nick was being prepared for discharge, Dr. Akintade estimated that 90 percent of his responses were accurate and appropriate. Donna was trained in all of the medical procedures still necessary to keep Nick alive, and would have the equipment and nursing assistance she needed at the house she had rented in Glen Burnie. "Home is always the best place for a person," Dr. Akintade was certain, and she felt that Nick would continue to improve and heal.

But no one could predict how far he would go. The doctors thought it was unlikely he would ever be the boy he was before he got shot in the head. He remained profoundly impaired—incapable of speaking, eating, walking, or even breathing on his own. For Donna, though, the fact that her son was aware and could communicate was an answer to her prayers. Each moment of interaction between mother and son was a blessing, a gift from God, and after all she had been through, her faith did not waver. She was certain God's plan for Nick was for continued improvement. She prayed:

Lord, I pray that I can care for him, that I won't do anything wrong. I pray for Nick's continued healing. Please, Lord, I hope that it is in Your plan for Nick to recover enough to have a useful life.

Part Three

THANKS

LEROY SCHAUER
From the Heart

Our gracious heavenly Father, we thank You for this day and for the strength and guidance You give us every day.

"Hello, I'm Reverend Schauer from the chaplain's office. I just stopped by to see how you're doing." Leroy Schauer grasps the hand of Henry Carlisle,* a patient on Nelson 5. Henry, forty-five, has a long, difficult medical history—nine years of gradually worsening cardiomyopathy, a dangerous weakening of the heart muscle. He has spent the last eleven months of that time hospitalized as his own heart wore down and he needed the medical support of a hospital to keep him alive. A former Baltimore firefighter, he is now awaiting a heart transplant. So far no suitable donor heart has come available.

Eleven months is a long time to be in the hospital but Henry says he's making the best of it. Friends and his pastor from the community come to visit. He often orders carryout food, delivered right to his hospital room. He is happy for the unexpected visit from Schauer, whom he's never met before, and bows his head as the minister prays for him:

> *We know how difficult it is for Henry to have gone through these past eleven months. We ask You to help him endure and we ask Your blessing for his family, who cares for him. We ask that his stay at the hospital be over soon and that he go home healthy.*

* Patient names in this chapter are changed for reasons of confidentiality.

Thanks

Henry speaks of patience and learning how to get along during his wait, but his words can't hide his frustration and weariness, his fear and anger. Roy Schauer hears the unexpressed despair and nods with empathy. "It's rough isn't it? I know a little about what you're going through. I know how tough it can get. I've had two heart transplants myself."

When Roy Schauer started feeling ill, back in the early 1980s, he was a vigorous man in his early forties, husband and father of two young sons, minister to the Washington United Church of the Deaf, in Takoma Park, Maryland, a Washington suburb. When illness struck, he had a conversation with God about what was happening to him, as he had done with every event in his life, small or large, for as long as he could remember.

Okay, God, what's the message? What do You have in mind for me, God? What's going on? Why is my health being threatened? Please, God, please, Jesus, help me through this difficult time.

At first Roy thought he'd had a heart attack. On Memorial Day 1982, he was cutting his parents' lawn at their northeast Baltimore home. Feeling tired, he suddenly realized he was dripping with sweat, and even when he sat and rested, he continued to sweat profusely and couldn't shake the fatigue. His wife, Carole, a nurse, was alarmed. Over Roy's protestations, she insisted that they go to a community hospital emergency room.

Roy was diagnosed with a heart attack and admitted to the hospital, where he ended up spending two weeks. He was treated with standard heart attack medications—lidocaine to correct an irregular heartbeat, nitroglycerin to dilate the blood vessels and relieve the pain in his chest. He and Carole both attended cardiac rehabilitation classes that addressed the causes of a heart attack and how to stay healthy with exercise, stress reduction, and lowering cholesterol through diet.

Later, when he was back home in Hyattsville, another Washington suburb, he consulted with Brandis Marsh, a cardiologist at the Washington Hospital Center. Dr. Marsh asked a lot of questions: Do you smoke? Do you drink? Do you have much stress in your life? The answers were generally negative. Tests of his heart's pumping efficiency were also done, and this doctor came to a different diagnosis. "I don't think you had a heart attack at all," he told Roy and Carole. "I think you had a heart infection and now have cardiomyopathy."

"What's cardiomyopathy?" Roy responded.

Carole knew. Although her specialty was psychiatric nursing, she remembered enough from her nursing courses to know that cardiomyopathy is a dangerous weakening of the heart muscle. Some patients stabilize and live relatively normal lives. But for many, the path is of continuing deterioration, and the damage to the heart is irreversible.

About fifty thousand Americans are stricken each year with cardiomyopathy, making it a relatively uncommon heart disease. But it often affects younger adults, unlike other forms of heart disease, and can progress rapidly. Half of all people diagnosed with cardiomyopathy are dead within five years of diagnosis. In most cases, the cause of this grave disease is unknown.

No one ever understood exactly what caused Roy Schauer's heart to begin to wear out when he should have been in the prime of his life. His doctors speculated that an infection started the deterioration. Roy had thought of himself as a healthy person, although when he looked back he realized that he always seemed to get hit hard by the childhood diseases and ended up missing more school than the other kids. When he was eight, he had polio, and although it was a mild case with no resulting paralysis, he ended up missing much of the third grade.

Thanks

Roy grew up in east Baltimore, just a few blocks from The Johns Hopkins Hospital. From time to time he would visit ill family members there. In those years, the main lobby was at the Broadway entrance, leading into the rotunda where The Divine Healer stands. When Roy thought of Hopkins, he thought of the statue of Christ. Healing and faith were intertwined in his mind. The imposing statue made a strong impression on the young boy, and sometimes he would ask his parents to take him to the hospital just to see it, to stand by it and absorb its energy. His faith was one of the strongest constants in his young life—he never doubted God and went to church happily with his parents every week. One grandfather was a Methodist minister, uncles and cousins were also in the ministry, and Roy grew up enjoying and appreciating the comfort and support of a strongly religious family. He felt a close personal relationship with God and Christ. From childhood on, the church was the focus of his life, and his communication with God was ongoing. *God, please help me with this test. God, there's a bully on the street.* God was a welcome part of every facet of his life.

When Roy was a teenager, his family moved to the north suburbs where his father delivered bread and counted among his customers some of the players from the city's new baseball team, the Baltimore Orioles. Roy graduated from high school in 1956 and pursued his interest in art, first attending a community college and then graduating from the Maryland Institute, College of Art, and teaching art in area junior high schools.

He enjoyed teaching but didn't feel it was his calling, and through a night job followed a growing interest in working with people who were hearing impaired. He was already proficient in sign language—his next-door neighbor was hearing impaired and had stimulated that interest. Roy took a class at a church for the hearing impaired when he was in high school. He was particularly interested when a hearing-impaired missionary addressed the congregation and "spoke" of her ministry. He felt a bond with the church members—he liked them and they liked him. Then, when a good friend who was also a teacher entered a seminary to study for the ministry, Roy felt a spark within himself. This was the path *he* should be following. He entered Wesley Seminary in Washington in 1969, with the assurance he had found his life's work, and that his ministry would somehow serve the needs of the hearing-impaired community.

Before and during his seminary years, Roy served as chaplain at Gallaudet College, a school for people who are hearing impaired. He also taught classes in sign language, and one of his students was Carole Herlyn, a twenty-two-year-old nurse from South Dakota pursuing her own interest in working with the hearing impaired. Before long she had an interest in the teacher as well. Shortly after he graduated from the seminary in 1970, Roy and Carole were married. He was appointed to a ministry in a DC–area United Methodist church. The congregation was not hearing impaired, but Roy continued to hold an afternoon church service for hearing-impaired people and to work at Gallaudet. In 1974 he was appointed to a full-time pastoral care position at the Washington United Methodist Church for the Deaf.

There, Roy attended to more than the spiritual needs of the members of his congregation. He frequently accompanied his parishioners to court to interpret for them, or made doctors' appointments for them, or went with them on medical visits. Within a few years he and Carole had two sons of their own, born in 1972 and 1976. It could be hectic, and there were times when he had the feeling his life was not his own. But he loved his work, and being a father came as naturally to him as anything he'd ever done. Not a day went by that Roy didn't acknowledge his blessings and thank God for them, and he couldn't conceive of life without the hope that faith brings.

In 1982, when he first learned his heart ailment was cardiomyopathy, Roy felt a little confused, a little frightened, but usually he was able to continue life as almost normal. Sometimes the thought would creep in—*will I live to see my kids grow up?*—but mostly he didn't figure death was an imminent possibility. He followed his doctor's advice and didn't do any strenuous work, no heavy lifting or running. He took digoxin every day to strengthen his heart and help it pump more efficiently. And for more than three years he remained fairly stable.

Roy didn't ask many questions about his condition; he was glad just to know it wasn't forcing him to curtail too much in his life. But Carole researched the medical literature and learned that it was just a matter of time before a patient with cardiomyopathy goes into congestive heart failure, with the heart having more and more difficulty pumping. The knowledge hovered over her—sometimes she could forget about it, but sometimes she felt like she was spending her life waiting for calamity. *God, what's coming, what's around the corner?* she asked, trying not to despair. *When will congestive heart failure come? How am I going to deal with all of this?*

In spring of 1985, there was a hint of trouble to come—a strange episode when Roy was attending a church conference on a college campus. Walking across the grounds, he suddenly realized someone was talking to him, on his right side, and he couldn't see him—he had lost half of his vision. A nurse at the conference diagnosed a possible migraine headache and advised Roy to take a nap. He'd never had a migraine before and was a bit frightened. But his vision returned after about a half hour, he finally did fall asleep, and felt back to normal when he awakened.

But Roy knew his health was deteriorating. He looked at his gaunt face in a new driver's license photo and felt like he was looking at a stranger. He'd catch a glimpse of his shadow and think, *Who is that stooped old man?* During a car trip to visit his sister in Connecticut in the fall of 1985, Roy began to feel very ill. He started out driving, but several hours into the six-hour trip, Carole took the wheel. By the time they reached their destination, he was beginning to have trouble breathing and felt terrible, with a total lack of energy. When he lay down in bed, he felt he was suffocating and couldn't breathe. He spent the night sitting up in bed, propped up with pillows, and the next morning he and Carole rushed home—to an emergency appointment with his cardiologist.

The doctor was alarmed as soon as he saw Roy. He sat him down in a wheelchair, wheeled him into the hospital admitting area, and had him admitted. *Things are falling apart fast,* Roy thought. Fear was beginning to creep in, but he still didn't appreciate the severity of his condition. In an era of lesser medical technology, his remaining time would have been numbered in weeks or months, at best.

"Things are not looking real good," Dr. Marsh told Roy and Carole the next day, but there wasn't much he could offer in the way of treatment. In one conversation she had alone with the doctor, Carole broke into tears as he told her of the possibility of sudden death from a heart that was failing the way Roy's was. Not only was the pumping mechanism impaired, but the electrical system, which keeps a healthy heart beating in a regular way, was debilitated and causing uncorrectable arrhythmias. Carole thought of the boys, eight and twelve at the time. "How on earth am I going to explain this to my children?" she wept. "One day their father looks fine, the next I have to tell them he might die at any moment." Dr. Marsh looked at her compassionately. "I've had the same trouble trying to tell you," he said.

Carole sought solace from quiet personal prayers. *God, I open myself to Your care. Please, merciful God, watch over Roy, he needs Your help right now.* Roy was so sick that his prayers were little more than inchoate phrases—*please, God . . . Heavenly Father . . . give me strength . . . I feel so weak.*

Several days later, days of gradual deterioration, Dr. Marsh came into Roy's room with a treatment possibility that elicited both hope and fear. "Roy needs a new heart," he said. "A heart transplant. No one is doing them here in Washington, but up the road in Baltimore,

Johns Hopkins is a transplant center. I think Roy is a good candidate and, quite frankly, it's his only chance for a normal life."

Carole went home that night feeling burdened with the weight of making a difficult decision—the transplant seemed like a dangerous, experimental procedure, but what was the alternative? A phone call from home in South Dakota compounded her anguish. Her brother had been seriously injured that day in a grain elevator accident. Pinned under concrete for hours, he ended up needing his leg amputated. Carole worried and grieved for him from afar, wishing she could be home with her younger brother but knowing she couldn't leave Roy. Even with the family crisis in South Dakota, her family helped her too—her aunt flew in to take care of the boys, and three weeks later her mother arrived to provide child care and emotional support.

The day after Marsh suggested a heart transplant, Carole and Roy decided this was their best hope, and Roy was transferred to Hopkins in an ambulance. An echocardiogram, a sound wave image of the heart, showed severely depressed ventricular function, the pumping activity of the heart. In a letter to Marsh, Kenneth Baughman, Hopkins chief of cardiology who evaluated Roy, described "a dilated cardiomyopathy of horrendous proportions."

"Reverend Schauer was rapidly accepted into the heart transplant program," Baughman wrote.

Roy arrived at Hopkins for his first transplant in early November 1985. He was a very sick man—sick not only from his disease but also from the treatment, as is often the case in serious disease. The medications to stabilize his arrhythmia caused nausea, vomiting, diarrhea, partial paralysis, and mental confusion. He was quickly moved from the medical unit to the ICU. His deteriorating status escalated him up the hierarchy for receiving a donor heart—he was classified as an emergency. He could not wait weeks or months for an organ to become available. He was going downhill fast.

From the Heart

God, I have faith You will get me through this. Please, God, I am a young man, surely it could not yet be my time to leave this world.

The first human heart transplant took place in 1967, performed by Dr. Christiaan Barnard in South Africa. That patient lived only eighteen days. For the next sixteen years, heart transplantation remained an experimental procedure, used only as a last resort for dying patients. The two biggest barriers to success were lack of donor organs and rejection of transplanted organs. The body recognizes the transplanted heart as foreign, and the immune system attacks it. But in 1983, two years before Roy's first transplant, the introduction of the drug cyclosporine toppled the rejection barrier and provided much greater chances of recovery for transplant patients.

Cyclosporine suppresses rejection, and considerably increases the odds of long-term survival after transplantation. Today about 2,300 heart transplants are done each year in the United States, and 70 percent of heart transplant recipients live at least five years. But a suppressed immune system is vulnerable to infections and other problems, including serious ones like cancer and kidney failure. With a heart transplant, Roy would look forward to a life of daily medications, potential side effects from the drugs, and frequent medical monitoring. In November 1985, as he waited in a hospital bed for a donor heart to become available, management of heart transplant patients was a new discipline with many unknowns.

The greatest unknown was whether a suitable heart could be found in time. Heart transplantation was such a novel procedure that there were precious few donor hearts available. As Roy waited, days turned into bleak November weeks, the hours counting down. Roy was so weak, his blood pressure so low, he couldn't always manage the walk to the bathroom in his hospital room. One day he fainted in the bathroom and came to with his head cradled by Lisa Loeb, one of the nurses on the unit. His low blood pressure caused the world to look bright, a glow on it. *She is my guardian angel,* Roy thought of

the nurse who seemed to have a halo around her, and their special relationship would continue through years of subsequent hospitalizations.

The staff tried to keep his spirits up. "After the transplant, you're
going to be doing things you haven't done for a long time," Lisa assured him. Even as compromised as he was, his faith and goodness
made a positive impression on everyone. "Thank you for referring
this absolutely delightful and deserving candidate to us for cardiac
transplantation," Baughman wrote to Marsh.

In his prayers, Roy tried to express his appreciation for the excellent care he was receiving and not to dwell on his precarious situation. *God, thank You for all the Lisas who tend to the needs of those who
are sick,* he prayed. *Give them patience and understanding, knowledge
and wisdom, compassion and strength. Amen.*

Through his own church, and church networks around the world,
prayer chains were in place, and a continuing stream of prayer focused on Roy Schauer's declining heart. Carole heard that people
were praying for Roy in South Dakota, in England, in Hyattsville, in
California, in churches for the hearing impaired around the country.
She felt bolstered by the spiritual attention, reinforced and uplifted by
the knowledge that the prayers of many others joined her own. But
sometimes it was difficult to squelch her dread. She saw Roy on a
precipice, sliding downhill fast. One day she looked at his chart and
saw the words "fading rapidly." He was losing weight, not always co-
herent. Crash teams assembled almost daily at his bed in the critical
care unit as one or another of his monitors signaled an alarm. But he
kept reviving.

Organs for transplantation are recovered on a nationwide basis
from patients who are brain dead—that is, their brains have ceased to
function and there is no hope of recovery, but with artificial support,
blood continues to circulate through their organs, which remain alive
and healthy. These brain-dead individuals are a source of living organs for a growing variety of patients—today, kidneys, livers, lungs,

corneas, skin tissue, hearts, and pancreases are all successfully recovered and transplanted. The organs are assigned to awaiting recipients according to a clear-cut protocol based on blood type compatibility and need. In accordance with the ethical protocol of transplantation, Roy and Carole never learned from whom his new heart came.

⌒

Wednesday, November 27, the day before Thanksgiving, was rough. Roy was weakening—each check of his vital signs, every few hours, showed he was getting worse. Carole, at Roy's bedside and alone in the waiting room, prayed, using a technique that always helped her feel close to God. She visualized herself in the most calming, centered place she could imagine—looking out her mother's bay window in South Dakota, gazing over a field of green growing corn. Prayer for her is a form of meditation, deep and soothing. *Please, God, help Roy get through one more day, help me get through one more day.*

In the afternoon, the doctor told Carole that he didn't think Roy would live through another day. She was crying in a waiting room with Roy's mother, feeling the worst had come, when Lisa, Roy's favorite nurse, stuck her head in the door. "Looks like we've got a heart," she announced, and suddenly the world was a different place.

The surgery, performed by Michael Borkon, one of Hopkins' cardiac surgeons, took about six hours. By the time Roy was prepped and in the operating room and the donor heart put in, it was Thanksgiving Day. *An exceptional day to be thankful,* Carole thought later, eating turkey and fixings with Roy's mother and the boys in the Hopkins cafeteria. Her brother had been released from the hospital the day before. Roy's surgery had gone smoothly, and his prognosis was guardedly optimistic.

How great and marvelous are the works of Your hand, O God.
Even in times of deep distress, You never leave us alone. My heart

leaps with joy and my heart sings praise to You. Thank You.
Thank You. Thank You, almighty God.

Roy's impressions waking up with a new heart were of a huge room, his bed in the center of it, tubes going in and out of him. Because the immune system is compromised by antirejection drugs, transplant patients recovering from surgery are kept in a specially ventilated isolation area with two full-time nurses. There was a stationary bike in the room and within days he was pedaling away, tubes and all. Despite his debilitated condition before surgery, he recovered quickly. Every day he felt a little bit better. Carole looked at him, pedaling on the bike, sitting up in bed eating, and rejoiced.

Roy was discharged from Hopkins fifteen days after the operation. He was dazzled by the slanting December sunlight as he walked out the door. Carole drove home to Hyattsville with both of them feeling that a new life was beginning. Roy was a little shaky but eager to get back to work, although he knew he would have to ease into it. A month after the surgery he saw Baughman, who was pleased with his progress. In his examination notes, Baughman said the post-operative course was "amazingly uncomplicated" and described Roy as "somewhat haggard but well-appearing."

In the next months, though, problems developed. In January an infection put Roy back in the hospital for two weeks. Inexplicably, even as his new heart pumped healthily, Roy sank into a depression. He would find himself dwelling morbidly on all the other things that could go wrong with his health. Still not strong enough to be working full-time, he spent many hours sitting in the living room, huddled in a corner, staring at the wall, feeling alone and isolated. Sometimes he would cry quietly. Everything seemed so difficult, and he felt so tired. His faith didn't waver but sometimes he felt forsaken—or verging on it. *Where are You, God?* Roy wanted to know. *Why can't this go more smoothly, why can't I be healed more quickly? Why does everything have to be so hard?*

Carole, exhausted and emotionally drained herself, couldn't help responding to the depression with anger. She raged internally: *He's been through all this crap, he almost died, he survived, I kept this family going, now he's lying on the couch and won't even eat lunch.* It was a hard time for both of them. Roy, feeling sorry for himself, felt sorry for Carole too, but was unable to reassure her, to resume equal partnership in the marriage. Depression is a common problem among heart transplant recipients. Roy sought treatment, and gradually, as he got back to work full-time, his spirits lifted, the pall of depression dissipated, and he and Carole were both able to enjoy life again.

Life was back to normal for the Schauers, but normal was different from before. Good health, once taken for granted, could never be a certainty. Carole felt that questions hung over every issue in their lives—will we be able to take a vacation, buy a car, renovate the kitchen? In general, the medical reports over the next years were encouraging—but the transplant and medications to support it took their toll, and Roy's life had a fragility he had to get used to living with. Sometimes his semiannual heart biopsies would reveal some rejection going on, and Baughman would increase the antirejection drugs, only to have to make further adjustments to address the side effects of the drugs. It was a constant juggling act.

By 1989, though, many of the problems were resolved. "I feel marvelous," Roy told Baughman at a routine followup exam. "My life is truly unrestricted." But new problems were looming. Through the years, he'd fought a battle with high cholesterol. It was successfully lowered by medication for a while, but was now beginning to threaten his new heart. An angiogram in December 1989 found that his coronary arteries were "no longer pristine." Eleven months later the test showed "accelerated atherosclerosis"—considerable clogging of the coronary arteries. It was an ominous sign—not uncommon in heart transplant patients, but not reversible. The only effective treatment was another transplant.

Roy and Carole were stunned. They couldn't believe this was

happening. Roy felt fine. But the doctors were telling them that his blood vessels were closing up, that he could expect to feel dizziness and shortness of breath, although there wouldn't be much pain, because his transplanted heart did not have the same sensory nerves as his own heart. He was put on the list for people awaiting heart transplants, once again to wait for a donor heart.

It was June 1991. William Baumgartner, the cardiac surgeon who was now seeing Roy, told him to pick up a beeper on the way home, so he could be paged and alerted immediately when a heart became available. Roy and Carole were eating dinner that evening when the beeper went off. "Oh, it's probably a false alarm or a mistake," Roy said. As he was looking at the beeper read-out, the phone rang. Carole picked it up. "It's Dr. Baumgartner," she said, handing the phone to Roy. "Are you sitting down?" Baumgartner began. "You'd better, because I think we've got a heart for you."

The experience couldn't have been more of a contrast to the transplant six years previously, when Roy was near death before a heart became available. This time he didn't even feel ill. He, Carole, and Andrew, their younger son, drove to Baltimore. Roy checked into Hopkins, and hours later Baumgartner removed his heart and put a new one in his chest. Once again, he was not told who had died to give him a heart. But a professional athlete from Baltimore had been in a fatal car crash that day, shortly after Roy was placed on the waiting list. He and Carole couldn't help believing that the dead athlete's heart now beat in his body.

Roy received his second new heart on Friday, June 21, 1991, and things went so smoothly that by Monday, Carole had decided to go ahead with plans for an oft-delayed kitchen renovation. In the coming days, she brought sample books with her when she visited Roy in the hospital, so he could consult about the new cabinets, appliances, and décor.

Roy felt blessed and humbled. People waited months and years for suitable organs to become available for transplant—many died waiting. Why had he been so lucky to get *two* new hearts? *Heavenly*

Father, I don't even know how to put my feelings into words, he prayed in thanksgiving. *I don't know what I did to deserve this, why You would put so much effort into providing for me. But thank You, God, thank You from the bottom of this healthy pumping heart, and I will try to be worthy of Your effort.*

Recovery was steady, but interrupted by a series of diverse medical problems—a perforated ulcer in his intestine, general fatigue, continuing high cholesterol, an infection in his right leg, a respiratory infection, the beginnings of kidney disease. When he was admitted to Hopkins in summer 1992 for a fever and cough after a trip to London, Baughman wrote in Roy's chart, "Clearly this is yet another life-threatening event in this patient's post-transplant history." Most of these continuing health problems could be attributed to the side effects of cyclosporine or prednisone, another drug Roy took to prevent rejection of his transplanted heart. Perhaps his most serious problem came after a family trip to the Grand Canyon in 1994. Horseback riding, he and Carole passed other horses going the opposite way on the same narrow trail, and Roy's leg was scraped by a plastic crate on the back of an oncoming horse. Continuing use of prednisone causes weakening of skin tissue, and Roy's leg was torn open. He was transported from the scene and treated in a hospital in Kingman, Arizona, but when he returned home he needed further treatment to repair the damage done. It was a very painful episode.

Roy realized by now that a bump that would cause no problem for most people resulted in at least a bruise and possibly much worse for him. Though he did heal from these injuries, recovery could be slow. He started feeling that his body was no longer his own, but was resigned to the continuing insults. *Oh, shoot, not again,* he thought, when things went wrong. And then he'd thank God that it wasn't worse and remind himself of how truly blessed he was.

Again and again, visiting patients at Hopkins who are waiting for transplants or recovering from transplant surgery, Roy Schauer feels fellowship and acceptance when he reveals that he has had two heart transplants himself. Sometimes, as when he saw Henry Carlisle, who had been waiting eleven months for a new heart, he feels twinges of guilt about his own good luck and wonders why he was so lucky. But more and more, as the years pass, the meaning is clear.

Dropping in on transplant patients on various units in the hospital, Roy remembers the high and low points of his own transplants— the declines leading to them, the climbs back to recovery, the succession of complications that brought him back into the hospital. Through some of it, he was too sick to remember much. But some images stick. "I've been on every one of these floors," he muses as he walks from one unit to another, "but I can't always remember when I was where."

During some of his hospitalizations, when he didn't have too many tubes in him and was relatively free to move around, he reacquainted himself with The Divine Healer. As he stood at the pedestal and gazed up at the serene figure, he visualized himself as a child in the same spot, remembering the feeling he'd had then of peace and faith, of being cared for. *Jesus, I never thought I'd be spending so much time here as a patient,* he thought, *but it sure is a comfort knowing You're still here for me.*

Now he usually comes to the hospital not as a patient but as a member of the adjunct chaplaincy staff. He will often stop in the rotunda for a silent moment with The Divine Healer, still as moved by the figure as he was when he was a boy. Then he moves into the chapel where he sits for moments more, his hands folded, his head bowed.

Please, God, be with me as I visit with patients, he prays. *In Your infinite wisdom, please give me the right thoughts, the right words to minister to them. Allow me to be of help to their families and to those providing their medical care, the doctors and nurses. Lord, please give me the right words to speak so that my visit will make a difference in their lives.*

From the Heart

Sometimes he is alone in the chapel, which is on the first floor of the hospital, tucked unobtrusively off the Children's Center lobby. Often others will come, pray, and go: relatives of patients; sometimes patients themselves, attached to an IV; visiting clergy; doctors, nurses. It is not unusual for someone to be weeping. This small hushed circular room has witnessed many moments of grief, as well as thanksgiving. Ten chairs are arranged around the perimeter, facing an altar backed by a mosaic wall. Soothing blue tiles edged with gold depict a pastoral scene—a small flock of sheep, a scattering of simple flowers. In staggered letters the words of the Twenty-third Psalm are inscribed: *The Lord is my shepherd, I shall not want. He maketh me to lie down in green pastures. He leadeth me beside the still waters. He restoreth my soul.*

After praying in the chapel and before visiting patients, Roy walks around and talks with some of his many acquaintances in the hospital. Some have sought his guidance and prayer for their own personal and health problems: a secretary who is struggling with putting her mother in a nursing home; a nurse whose son is in a drug treatment program; another secretary personally suffering the progressive debilitation of ALS (Lou Gehrig's disease).

His full-time ministry is now at Corkran Memorial United Methodist Church, in Temple Hills, Maryland, but he usually manages at least a day a week at Hopkins, fifty miles away. To him, this second ministry is a continuing reminder of how the positives of change brought on by illness can outweigh the negatives. A failing heart is not something he would have chosen, but he thanks God for the way it has enhanced his ministry and brought him in contact with a group of patients whose difficult problems he can truly understand. His pastoral care with his own congregation is inclined to help more with medical problems than other ministers: he often visits sick parishioners at their homes or at the hospital; sometimes he accompanies congregation members on medical visits. He can give advice and guidance, practical tips and mental preparation with the certainty of one who has been there. For example, a woman wants to know what to expect from the heart biopsy her doctor scheduled her for. Roy can tell her plenty—he's had at least seventy heart biopsies in the past fifteen years.

Sitting on the edge of the bed, clasping hands with Ellen Lowell, a Nelson 5 patient who has had pancreas and kidney transplants, and her adult daughter, Roy's prayer offers a message of hope:

> *Our gracious heavenly Father, we are most thankful for You and for Your guidance and presence in our lives. Without You, we never would be able to make it. We ask that You open Your heart to this family, that You bring healing, and that You bless the doctors and nurses in their healing mission.*

Ellen speaks honestly and emotionally of the battle she fights every day, of how her faith sometimes wavers, how she gets angry at God. "But I know I wouldn't be here without Him," she adds quickly. "The physician will dress the wound but God will heal it. It is not for us to ask why, is it?"

Roy speaks from his personal experience when he answers. "After my first transplant, I remember questioning, why did this happen to me? And then the second time it hit me—there's a reason for my being here. There's a reason this has happened to me."

He remembers another patient having a difficult time, a teenage girl who was awaiting a kidney transplant. She was Jewish, but glad for support from a clergyman of any faith, and they prayed together. But she was bitter and suffering with the "why me?" question. Roy comforted her as best he could, telling her a little about Rabbi Harold Kushner's book *When Bad Things Happen to Good People*. As he left her bedside, he wished he could have done more. He went downstairs to the chaplain's office and gathered his mail. In his box was a letter with a ten-dollar bill in it. Feeling that the money was a sign from God, he walked down the corridor to the gift shop, bought the Kushner book, and had a nurse deliver it to the girl.

What's the message, God? Roy asks the question often, sometimes standing at the foot of The Divine Healer, who has become such a familiar figure from his many trips to Hopkins. The answers, he has found, usually come in hindsight, but the lesson that seems to be continually reinforced is that for him, and for everyone, so much is out of his own hands. In the expressive sign language of the hearing impaired, he throws up his hands—the sign for giving up. But he is not really giving up, just acknowledging that the final choices are in the hands of God. *Okay, God, it's up to You, I can't do anything more about it.* And then he will pray, a prayer of faith and trust:

O Lord, You are the creator and sustainer of life. You love us more than we know and love ourselves. Your love is never failing. Even as we journey through the valley of the shadow of death, You are there. Give to us who struggle to hold on to life the strength to endure, and the knowledge that You are near. Into Your hands we put our trust.

MARVIN FOXWELL

A Chaplain's Blessing

Please dear Lord, let my husband feel better.
Amen.

Patricia Foxwell wiped away a tear as she finished writing her short prayer in the book at the Christ statue. A few buildings away, her husband, Marvin, lay in a hospital bed, sicker than she'd ever seen him. It terrified her. They'd been together since she was little more than a child—she was sixteen and he was nineteen when they married. They heard all the warnings then about teenage marriages not making it, but here they were, forty-two years later, proving that young love can grow into mature lifelong devotion and companionship.

They'd come to Hopkins from their home in North Carolina. She and Marvin had lived there only four years, happy years of waking each morning to the shimmering view of the Perquimans River outside their many-windowed bedroom wall. On a clear day she could see beyond the wide river to the small town of Hertford, the same town just south of the Virginia/North Carolina border where she and Marvin exchanged their wedding vows.

Marvin Foxwell and Patricia Pegram grew up across town from each other in Portsmouth, Virginia, just up the coast from Hertford. Their fathers worked together in the same shipyard in the Tidewater city. They met at a high school football game and then double dated—Marvin was with Pat's identical twin sister Priscilla; Pat was with another boy. Something clicked almost right away; before the end of that first date, the twins switched dates.

The Pegram twins were restless teenagers, unhappy at home, bored at school, and wanting to move on with their lives. Within months, Priscilla and her boyfriend ran away to South Carolina, where minors didn't need parental consent for marriage. Pat and Marvin went with them and thought marriage looked like a good idea. With her sister gone, Pat felt terribly lonely at home. She and Marvin told their parents they wanted to get married, but didn't want to go all the way to South Carolina. Their parents thought they were young, but didn't object, and their dads went with them and signed for them in Hertford. Back in Portsmouth, the young couple lived with Marvin's parents for about a month, then rented an apartment of their own. Pat worked for a factory that made Christmas trees and ornaments, Marvin for a factory that made industrial uniforms.

Before long the girls came—Theresa in 1957, Kimberly five years later. Pat was just seventeen when Theresa was born, but she loved being a mother, and Marvin was a good provider. He started moving up in the company, and she could be a full-time mom. They bought their first house before Kim was born, a brick rancher in Chesapeake, Virginia, around the bay from Portsmouth.

Patricia felt God was good to her. She hadn't had a strong religious upbringing but she wanted to make sure God knew how thankful she was for her healthy children, her good marriage, Marvin's devotion and tenderness. She started going to a small Presbyterian church in the community and over a period of time felt herself open to God's grace and the divinity of Christ. She experienced no single "born-again" event but felt secure and certain in her faith. Marvin had felt strong Christian beliefs since he was a teenager, and he felt supported and sustained by being a regular member of a congregation. For years they went with the girls to Sunday morning services and Wednesday evening Bible study. Pat called it a midweek refueling. She and Marvin both felt their faith was solid and unshakable. But life was good, and so far their faith hadn't much been tested.

⌒

Theresa and Kim grew up, married, each had two children of her own. Pat was a grandmother when she was only forty-two. The girls and their families stayed in the Tidewater area, and they remained close, with Pat providing a fair amount of the child care for her grandchildren. Marvin continued rising in his company, a steady progression to plant manager, general manager, vice president. His quick intelligence, affable manner, and knowledge of the company served him well. When a European firm with plants around the world bought the company, travel became part of Marvin's job—Germany, Switzerland, England. He enjoyed the travel at first, but began to find it fatiguing.

As they moved into middle age, Pat and Marvin started experiencing a few health problems. Marvin had his gallbladder removed in 1985 and didn't heal as quickly as he should have from the abdominal incision. The doctor told him this was the way his body responded to surgery, and he should keep it in mind if he was ever operated on again. Pat found out she had high blood pressure and suffered a "mini stroke" in 1997. She learned then that she'd had a previous stroke, without knowing it. She was hospitalized at Maryview Hospital in Portsmouth, and five hours later Kim was brought in to give birth to her second child. At least the timing turned out to be convenient, with Pat and Kim in the hospital at the same time, and the diagnosis was a wake-up call for Pat to modify her diet and start a regular exercise program.

The symptoms of the tumor that brought Marvin to Hopkins began around Christmastime 1998 and were subtle. At first he thought it was a cold or the flu, producing a bad backache. For the first time in years, he and Pat broke their tradition of Christmas morning with their children and grandchildren. He was so uncomfortable that they drove home Christmas Eve from Theresa's, where they had planned to spend the night. The kids visited the next day, but Marvin felt he was just going through the motions, not feeling well enough to celebrate Christmas.

A day later he waited two hours to be seen in a neighborhood health center and was diagnosed with a kidney infection and bronchitis. A few days on antibiotics helped, but just after New Year's the clinic called and suggested he have a followup X ray. He took the first films to James Cochran, his internist in Portsmouth, who saw a suspicious spot and ordered a CAT scan. The spot showed up at the very bottom of the scan, which had primarily looked at Marvin's lungs. Another scan was taken, aiming lower in his abdomen for a better view.

On January 10, Pat and Marvin heard the results together from Cochran. As soon as Pat saw the doctor, perched on the end of his desk, she knew he didn't have good news. Marvin, feeling much better physically, was also anxious. "It's a good thing we looked further down," the doctor told them. "It looks like there's a tumor on your pancreas."

Pat couldn't believe it. The word "tumor" sounded so frightening. "He hasn't even been that sick," she protested.

"There are usually no signs until it's pretty far along," Cochran said.

"Are you telling me he has cancer?" Pat demanded.

"There's a tumor on his pancreas, and you should get it looked at right away," the doctor answered. He referred them to Mark Lawson, a gastroenterologist in the area.

Lawson saw them the next day. "It's obvious there's something in there and it has to come out," he told Pat and Marvin after he looked at the scans and examined Marvin. He said he could biopsy the tumor himself but suggested they find a surgeon who specialized in operating on pancreatic tumors. He didn't have any doubt where they should go. "The best person in the country is Dr. John Cameron at Johns Hopkins in Baltimore."

Lawson agreed with Cochran that the diagnosis was a bleak one. "It is unlikely that the [mass] represents a . . . benign process," he wrote in his clinic notes. Pat and Marvin were bewildered and frightened—they hardly knew what a pancreas was. But they learned all too quickly the discouraging prognosis for pancreatic cancer—less than 5 percent of patients live more than five years after diagnosis. More than half are dead within six months of learning they have the disease.

When Lawson called Cameron's office, he was able to schedule an appointment for Marvin in three days, on Friday, January 22. Pat and Marvin weren't even sure if their health insurance would cover treatment in Baltimore, but they didn't care. They had a substantial amount of savings in the bank and mutual funds. Neither had any interest in the money without the other to share it with. If this is what it would take to get the best possible medical care for Marvin, they would do it.

The day before they left for Baltimore and their first appointment at Hopkins, they drove the couple of miles from home across the river into Hertford. They had dinner at the café in Hertford and drove around the block to the little house where they had exchanged their wedding vows. Now a private residence, it was once one of several marriage chapels in the area that served couples who traveled from nearby states with more stringent marriage requirements.

In the decades that had passed since they were married, they had enjoyed contentment and satisfaction and good fortune together. But now they feared what the future might hold. They sat in their car with the license plate MARV&PAT in front of the onetime wedding chapel, held hands, and prayed:

Pat: *Please, God, if it is Your will, please spare Marvin. Please let it not be cancer. Lord, watch over Marvin.*
Marvin: *Lord, if it be Your will that I come through this, I want to remain here with my family and enjoy my later years with them. Please, Lord, let that happen.*

Surgeons call the pancreas the "rattlesnake" of the abdomen because it is such a difficult organ to operate on, delicate in texture and closely connected to other organs and blood vessels. The pancreas performs two essential functions: it produces enzymes to aid digestion and it manufactures insulin, which is needed to metabolize glucose, the body's primary source of energy.

John L. Cameron, chief of surgery at The Johns Hopkins Hospital, has had as much experience with pancreatic surgery as any other surgeon in the world. The customary procedure to remove a diseased pancreas is called a Whipple, after the Columbia University surgeon who devised it in the 1930s. Specifics of a Whipple vary, depending on the size and location of the tumor. The classic Whipple removes most of the pancreas, the upper section of the small intestine (duodenum), the gallbladder, and the bile duct, the connection to the liver. Enough pancreas is left to continue producing insulin, and the gastrointestinal tract is reconnected so the patient will be able to eat and digest normally.

Pancreatic cancer is aggressive and usually not responsive to chemotherapy or radiation. The Whipple offered most patients their only chance of survival. But the operation itself, involving so many organs and blood vessels, is very risky and at one time was associated with a high mortality rate. In 1969, when Cameron, then chief surgical resident at Hopkins, performed his first Whipple, national survival rates were discouraging—one in four patients died during or soon after surgery. At that point, the procedure was falling into disfavor, done less and less, as increasingly the risk of death was seen as too high. When a Whipple was done, it was usually seen as the patient's last chance.

To Cameron, the Whipple offered a group of patients their only hope for life. He became consumed with perfecting the operation, increasing the survival odds, making it viable. Over the years, the challenge became his life's work. By the time Marvin Foxwell came to see him, Cameron had a national reputation for his success with the procedure and performed as many as five Whipples a week. His years of painstaking refinement had paid off—the mortality rate for his patients during or soon after surgery was less than 2 percent, a number that could be matched at only a couple of other hospitals nationwide. Many patients came from much farther than the Foxwells to avail themselves of Cameron's experience and expertise.

When Cameron examined Marvin Foxwell, he agreed with the Virginia doctors that they were probably looking at a malignancy. "But it's fairly small, and we caught it early, and you'll be out of here in eight or nine days," he reassured Pat and Marvin. In his clinic notes he described Marvin as "a healthy guy" and a good candidate for a Whipple. Surgery was scheduled for January 29.

In the week they were home before the surgery, Pat found out their insurance would cover 80 percent of their medical expenses in Baltimore. That was a relief. She made reservations to stay at a Baltimore hotel during the postoperative period—it was important to her and Marvin that she be close at hand through the entire experience. Kim came with them to Baltimore; the plan was that Theresa, taking care of Kim's children back in Virginia, would come up in several days to be with her father and Kim would return home and take care of the children.

Surgery would take at least six hours, Cameron told them. Restless and frightened, Pat and Kim decided to explore the hospital a little. They found the chapel, and Pat felt tremendously soothed just sitting there. *Please, Lord, let it not be cancer,* she prayed. *Please let us get through this day.* A song that she loved popped into her mind and she hummed quietly,

One day at a time, sweet Jesus, *Yesterday's gone, sweet Jesus,*
That's all I'm asking from You. *And tomorrow may never be mine,*
Just give me the strength to do *Lord, help me today, show me the*
 every day *way,*
What I have to do. *One day at a time.*

The surgery proceeded smoothly. Once in the abdomen, Cameron could see that the pancreas was inflamed. On the chance that it was this pancreatitis that had shown up as a tumor, he had the CAT scan reviewed. The radiologist confirmed there was definitely a mass in the head of the pancreas. Most likely, the inflammation was due to the tumor. The pancreatitis made the organ even more fragile than usual to handle. But Cameron has done this procedure so many times, he knows the feel of the tissue in his hand, the exact amount of pressure needed on the scalpel to dissect the blood vessels from the organs, precisely where to aim his knife to avoid nicks into blood vessels or organs. (Such nicks, along with leaking from the rejoined parts of the digestive system, were responsible for the previous high death rate from this operation.) Cameron meticulously worked his way to the walnut-size tumor and lifted it out with the surrounding tissue. As soon as it was out of the body, it was sent to the pathology lab, only a few yards down the hall.

After praying in the chapel, Pat and Kim went back to the waiting room. They saw patient representatives and doctors in surgical scrubs talking to other families, but no one had news for them. Finally, a patient rep called their name and then asked them to step into a private room. "The doctor will be here in a few minutes," she said.

Pat and Kim were terrified. In their hours of waiting, they hadn't seen anyone else taken to a private room. "Being in this room is not good," Kim wailed. "I think they lost Dad in surgery. Here we are, all alone."

Pat tried to console her daughter and squelch her own fears. "We're not alone," she said. "God is with us." But Kim was panicking and Pat felt the same way. It seemed an hour but was more like five minutes before Cameron showed up.

Cameron was smiling. "There is no cancer," he said. He was surprised himself—he had expected the tumor to be malignant, but the analysis revealed it was a cystic neoplasm, a benign tumor. The frozen section pathology report described it as a "simple cyst lined by columnar epithelium [a type of cell] without atypia." Little is known about what causes such a tumor, but it is likely that if left alone it eventually would have become malignant. And the pancreas was so inflamed that the extensive surgery was needed, even though the organ was cancer free.

Pat and Kim were so relieved they couldn't speak. They hugged each other and wiped tears off each other's cheeks. Cameron told them Marvin's pancreas was so fragile that he might have to remove it all, leaving no means of producing insulin. "He'll probably be a diabetic," he said, "but let me go back and see if I can save anything. We should be done in a couple of hours."

The hours went by with no report, and Pat and Kim felt their anxiety growing again. Pat started pacing. "Kim, I think there's something wrong," she said after about four more hours of waiting. She asked the patient representative what was going on, and the rep checked and said that Marvin was out of surgery and in the intensive care unit. "Why can't I see him?" Pat demanded. "When can I see my husband?"

"They're having an emergency in the ICU right now," the rep told her. "No one can go in there."

"Maybe Dad is the emergency," Kim said, and they were both shaken by this thought. After several more anxious minutes, a nurse confirmed that Marvin was indeed the emergency. His blood pressure had dropped precipitously, but he was improving. "We're working on him now," she said. "We're not sure what went wrong, but we're getting the pressure back up, and you can see him in about a half hour."

Finally, Pat was at her husband's bedside, holding his hand. She couldn't believe how bad he looked—swollen all over, hooked up to so many machines, his skin cold to the touch. *Please God, don't take him from me, don't let me lose him,* she prayed as she clutched his hand. On a ventilator, he couldn't talk and Pat couldn't tell if he saw her or not. When his eyes were open they seemed vacant, but once or twice she felt he was looking at her. And every now and then, he would squeeze her hand, a good solid squeeze. Before she and Kim left him to go back to the hotel for a few hours of sleep, she lifted his hand and pressed it against her teary cheek. "Now listen, Marvin," she said, "if anything goes wrong, you fight. You fight as hard as you can."

Kim had called her sister while waiting to get into the ICU, and Theresa packed up her daughters and jumped in the car to make the six-hour drive to Baltimore. She arrived at the hotel in the middle of the night, and in the morning wanted to see her dad as soon as she could. Pat, not yet ready to return to the hospital, said she would stay with her granddaughters while Theresa and Kim visited their father. It occurred to her that Marvin might wonder why she wasn't there. In fact, when he saw Theresa, all he could think of was that she had come to Baltimore hurriedly because Pat had another stroke. He couldn't talk, couldn't ask, but the nurses could see he was agitated. One put a pencil in his hand and held up a clipboard for him to write on. "Is my wife OK?" he wrote in shaky letters. His daughters reassured him that Pat was fine and would visit soon. Later that morning when Pat arrived at the hospital, she cried when the nurse showed her the note. "I will keep this note forever," she said.

Later, Cameron would describe Marvin's recovery from surgery as "a very complicated and extended course." He remained in the ICU and then in an intermediate ICU more than a week, with continuing low blood pressure and low-grade fever. But soon the breathing tube was removed, he began working with a respiratory therapist and could get up out of bed. Cameron had managed to leave enough pancreas in him to continue producing insulin, so that was good news. But then another crisis—the surgical incision reopened, and he was rushed back into surgery to have it repaired.

The repair was successful, but Marvin was not doing well. He and

Pat remembered his gallbladder operation nearly fifteen years ago, and how he had taken longer than expected to recover from that. This time, it was soon clear that the predicted ten-day hospital stay would be much longer than that. After the second surgery Marvin continued to run low-grade fevers. He was depressed, making little effort to walk around, an important activity for patients recovering from major surgery. He still was not eating and had to be sustained through intravenous feeding; for the first couple of weeks after the Whipple, it was unclear whether an adequate connection had been made between his digestive organs to allow normal digestion.

Pat didn't want to leave him. But it was draining, staying in the hospital room all day and evening, shuttling back to the hotel for a few hours of sleep, then back to the hospital early enough to see the doctors on their morning rounds. In her talks with the nurses, she learned of the Marburg Pavilion, the Hopkins unit with hotel-like amenities, a gourmet kitchen, and rooms large enough to bring in a bed for a spouse. Accommodations on Marburg cost more than the rate for rooms elsewhere in the hospital, and insurance policies do not cover the difference. (While medical care is the same in all Hopkins units, insurers do not pay for the extra amenities on Marburg.) In deciding to move to Marburg, Pat and Marvin had the same reaction they'd had when they first decided to come to Baltimore. Money didn't matter. Pat was paying for the hotel anyway, and the cost for the Marburg room wouldn't be much more than that. They would dip into their savings and both move to Marburg.

The Marburg Pavilion was established in 1996 to provide extra comforts for hospital patients who were willing to pay for them. Hopkins is one of a growing number of big-city medical centers nationwide with such a unit. Sports heroes, movie stars, foreign royalty, nationally known politicians—the rich and famous make up much of the population of this floor. But there are plenty of "common" folk like the Foxwells who are also willing to pay the cost.

The surroundings were well appointed and unhospital-like. In the hall were herringbone hardwood floors, oriental rugs, and French Provincial antiques that Pat found out had been owned by famous Hopkins surgeon William Halsted, one of the hospital's founding physicians. In the rooms, sliding wood panels covered the medical equipment behind the bed. Every room had its own fax machine, safe, computer hookup, VCR, and premium cable TV channels. Pat and Marvin thought it was funny that the Saudi Arabian news channel was among the TV selections—in deference to oil-wealthy Arabs who were treated at Marburg. The food was outstanding—although Marvin wasn't eating yet. Most important, it was great for Pat to have her own bed in the room with Marvin.

But gleaming floors and handsome furniture couldn't disguise the fact that Marvin was having a slow and difficult recovery. Cameron was upbeat and positive, reassuring Marvin and Pat that this was just a prolonged recuperation, that nothing life-threatening was going on. "Work with me, Mr. Foxwell," he would say. "Hang in there."

It wasn't easy. Days dragged into weeks; Marvin had been in the hospital for more than a month and was still not eating, barely ambulatory, depressed and despondent. He had drains in his side that were uncomfortable. One day he went out for tests, thinking that the drains were finally going to come out, but returned to the room with the tubes intact. "I'm never going to get out of here," he mumbled to Pat, and he was crying. Karen Whittaker, one of the nurses on the floor, went to the gift shop and came back with a little guardian angel pin. "Maybe this will help," she said, and pinned it to his IV pole.

The guardian angel made Pat realize what would help her, and maybe Marvin too. With all her anxiety, she had not thought to request pastoral assistance. "Is there anyone here who can pray with us?" she asked Karen, who called the chaplain's office. The next day the Reverend Stephen Mann was at Marvin's bedside for a prayer session that continued nearly every day for the rest of his hospitalization.

Stephen Mann, director of the hospital's chaplaincy staff, doesn't pray with patients as much as he once did. Hopkins chaplain since 1994, Mann has seen his job evolve into primarily administrative, research, and teaching duties, while his assistants take on more of the clinical responsibilities. But he tries to cover the spiritual needs of the patients on several units, and Marburg 3—where many patients are far from home and their personal clergy—is one of them. When he stopped by to see the Foxwells, he hoped he could provide the religious dimension they needed to make Marvin's prolonged hospital stay more bearable.

Before he prays, Mann talks with the people he is praying for and with, and uses their specific words to frame his prayer. The language in his prayers is usually more colloquial than conventionally spiritual—his view is that petitions are acceptable to God in one's own vernacular without spiritual "prettification." He also thinks it's important that people realize that their prayers reach God as clearly as the prayers of a clergyperson.

Mann could see Marvin and Pat were distressed about the complications that had developed and anxious about his prognosis. Spared cancer, they feared Marvin would never recover from the surgery. It was also clear to the chaplain that Marvin was as concerned about how Pat was handling this ordeal as she was for his health. At their first meeting, he visited with them for nearly an hour and could see them both relaxing. It was a relief to Pat and Marvin to have someone in the room who wasn't there to poke or prod him, or take him somewhere for a test, or take his blood pressure or temperature. From the first, they felt comfortable with the chaplain. His being there was a personal reminder of the Lord's presence. Before Mann left, he grasped hands with the Foxwells and prayed.

God, Marvin and Pat are in a period of much uncertainty and we pray that You will help them know that You are present in the midst of this uncertainty. Please help them draw upon their spiritual resources and utilize the comfort of knowing You are present and they are not alone. Please help Mrs. Foxwell get the rest and comfort she needs. Please help Mr. Foxwell continue to heal from surgery and get his strength back. Brighten his outlook so he can be rid of the depression that is dragging him down. Thank You, Lord.

The season was about to change, mild, spring-promising March days that Pat would get whiffs of on her brief forays out of the hospital. Marvin was moving around a little more, feeling better, but still too sick to leave the hospital. She couldn't believe how long they had been in Baltimore—they had settled into Marburg 309 and sometimes it felt like they'd been there forever. Staying on Marburg was comfortable—she was enjoying the meals, putting on some weight from too many beef Wellington dinners and cheesecake and chocolate truffle desserts. One night in mid-March, when they were watching a movie on the VCR in the room, Marvin reached over to Pat, sitting in a chair next to his bed, and took her hand.

"Honey, let's pretend this is our second honeymoon," he said.

"We might as well," Pat replied. "We deserve a second honeymoon after all this."

Every morning when the attending physicians, residents, and medical students came on their rounds, Pat would fire questions at them. When is this drain coming out? Why does he still need oxygen, why haven't his lungs cleared of congestion? Why does it still hurt him so much to walk? "Hon, you're going to run all the doctors off," Marvin told her gently.

Visits with the chaplain and trips to the statue and chapel helped decrease Pat's anxiety and get her through the days. The first time she saw the statue, when Marvin was still so sick, she burst into tears. She knelt at the base and reached out to rub the smooth foot. She *had* to touch Him—it was almost a compulsion. Rising and reading through the poignant prayers of others in the nearby book, she was touched by the stories, sometimes heartbreaking, that she could piece together from the messages. She had to leave her own prayer. The statue became a regular stop in her travels around the hospital, and she wrote in the book more than once, giving thanks as Marvin finally started to recover.

Thank You, Lord, for my husband's recovery. Please continue to watch over him. Amen.

—MARCH 14, 1999

Pat knew that Reverend Mann could tell when she was having a bad day, and she was comforted by his regular visits and prayers. He seemed to know just what to say, when to promise that things would get better, when to offer consolation for the current situation. To Pat, the chaplain was a blessing in her and Marvin's lives. He sat with her and looked at her collection of grandchildren pictures, heard the stories about the children, about home on the river in North Carolina. His prayers were often very specific and pragmatic. *Please, Lord, let this tube be ready to come out.* And as March came to an end and Dr. Cameron was promising discharge soon, Mann prayed, holding Pat's hand, *Please keep the way clear for Marvin to be discharged. They've been away from home for a long time, and they're ready to go now, if it's possible. And if for some reason that doesn't happen, please give them continued patience to wait for the right time to go.*

In addition to the slow healing of his incision, part of what kept Marvin in the hospital so long was concern about whether his digestive tract was functioning properly. From IV and tube feedings, he had progressed to clear liquids and then solid food, but was still having trouble holding food down. On the morning of the last Friday in March, Dr. Cameron said if Marvin could keep down two liters of fluid through the weekend, he could go home on Monday. Pat and Marvin thought he'd made it—and were dismayed when he threw up Sunday afternoon. But when the doctor saw him Monday morning, he said things looked pretty good. He was discharging Marvin. It was time to go home.

They decided to make the trip by car, with Theresa's husband, Russell, driving the six hours between Baltimore and Theresa's home in Chesapeake, where Marvin would do his first round of recuperating out of the hospital. The drive was stressful. Marvin's incision oozed blood. He couldn't believe how weak and helpless he felt. But it was still great to be out of the hospital, and Cameron assured them on the phone that the bleeding was not a problem. After a checkup three weeks after discharge, Cameron wrote in his clinic note, "The patient looks terrific . . . He is doing great, eating better, and I think he has made excellent progress." A CAT scan done that day showed a digestive system on its way to full recovery.

⌒

Full recovery came slowly, but it did come. A year after his operation, Marvin still sported an angry-looking wound on his belly from the incision, but it no longer caused pain or discomfort. His diet was back to normal, with pills supplying the digestive enzymes his pancreas no longer produced. There were no signs of diabetes. He gradually got back to work, but hadn't resumed full time and maybe never would. He was sixty-two, and the idea of early retirement was beginning to look more and more attractive. His medical experience— the brush with cancer, the long, slow recovery—made Marvin and Pat both appreciate the time they had with each other, with their daughters and their families, other friends and relatives. *I'd never have wished this and it was a hard way to learn,* Pat thought, *but now I know what's really precious in life.* Their prayers and the hand of God, they were very sure, had amplified the considerable skill of the surgeon. In their followup visits to Hopkins, they always stopped for a prayer in the chapel and at the statue, to leave a prayer of thanks. For Pat, the reminder of what they had been through was no further than her husband's belly:

A Chaplain's Blessing

Lord, this time I'm coming to You and giving thanks for Your blessings, and Lord, Marvin is right here with me. Thank You, Lord, so much for all of Your strength and all of Your help when at times, Lord, I just didn't know what to do. Most of all, Lord, I thank You for keeping Marvin here with me. Whenever I doubt, I just look at his badly scarred stomach and touch it and say thank You, Lord. Amen.

LILLIE SHOCKNEY

Prayer for a Mother,
Prayer for a Daughter

*Dear Lord, don't let my mother have what I had.
God, please shed Your grace over her and protect
my mom from this awful disease.*

In a pale lavender-walled radiology examining room in the Johns Hopkins Outpatient Center, Charmayne Dierker steps up to the X-ray machine and opens her hospital gown, exposing her breast to place it in the machine.

"We'll give you tassels later, Mom," says her daughter, Lillie Shockney, observing the procedure from behind a protective shield in the room.

Charmayne winces silently as the compression paddles move together, smashing her breast between them, spreading the tissue to provide the best possible view. At seventy-two, she is a tiny woman, and though the machine has been lowered to her level, she feels like she's stretching to reach it. In her self-effacing way, she apologizes to the radiology technician for her own discomfort. "I know all you're trying to do is save my life."

Like so many women, she is here because she felt a lump in her breast. She went through the same procedure six months ago when she felt a similar lump. Then, the biopsy following the mammogram removed the lump and revealed it was benign. Now it seems to have recurred, and she is worried—as is her daughter, despite her jokes.

Thanks

This is familiar territory for Lillie—offering guidance, support, humor when she can slip it in, and sometimes prayer to women undergoing diagnostic and treatment procedures for breast cancer. As education and outreach director of the Johns Hopkins Breast Center, she is often in the position of holding hands to provide moral support, facilitating referrals to the next level of care, answering frightened questions. But it's different when it's your own mom. A few years ago, Lillie and Charmayne formed an organization called Mothers Supporting Daughters with Breast Cancer. Sometimes, though, it's the other way around—sometimes daughters have to support mothers.

Now, as Charmayne's breast is flattened for the mammogram, Lillie bows her head and utters a silent prayer. *Please, God, give Mom the strength to endure whatever treatment she needs. Please help us all endure what's ahead.*

～

It will turn out that Charmayne's lump is benign, merely fibrocystic tissue, what radiologist Rachel Brem laughingly calls the "gristle" of the breast. It's a relief for everyone, for this is a family that has personally known cancer—Charmayne had uterine cancer years ago; Frank, Lillie's dad, was more recently treated for prostate cancer; Lillie's husband, Al, lost his mother to lung cancer; and Charmayne's father died of prostate cancer. Lillie's work for the Breast Center takes her all over the sprawling hospital, and the next time she passes through the Broadway lobby she will pause at the foot of The Divine Healer for a quick prayer of thanks.

Oh, God, You have once again enlightened our lives by giving us an opportunity to appreciate how precious good health is and never take it for granted. Thank You for sparing my mom from becoming a "club member" with me. Though I know she possesses the strength and courage to endure such a diagnosis, I'm pleased that she can redirect that energy into helping other women who are newly diagnosed.

The statue is an old friend. Lillie first met Him when she was a girl of thirteen. She already knew she wanted to be a nurse. She'd known that when she was barely more than a toddler, dressed up in a nurse's uniform, holding her bandaged doll for a photo she and her mom both still like to look at. It was the experience at age thirteen that convinced her she wanted to be a *Hopkins* nurse.

Lillie had been sick for three days, with nausea, vomiting, and intense pain in her abdomen. At the family home, a 360-acre dairy farm on Maryland's Eastern Shore, her mother worried and suffered with her for only a day or two before she took her to the family doctor in nearby Chestertown. He diagnosed a urinary tract infection and prescribed an antibiotic. Charmayne didn't say anything in the doctor's office, but driving home, Lillie, sick as she was, could hear her mother muttering, "I don't think that's what it is, I think he got it wrong." Terrified, Lillie was afraid to ask her mother what she did think the problem was. When she got sicker the next day her mother took her back to the doctor who this time diagnosed appendicitis.

Lillie's parents didn't want her to be operated on in the local hospital. Her father, Frank, had had an association with The Johns Hopkins Hospital for years, since his brother was treated there for a badly broken arm. Charmayne had been treated at Hopkins for migraines when she was a young woman. The family had formed a bond with a group of Hopkins doctors who met for decades every Thursday morning during goose-hunting season in the farm's abundant preserves. Soon Frank and Charmayne were driving Lillie the ninety miles to Baltimore, where she was quickly moved into an operating room for an emergency appendectomy.

It was a snowy week in January 1965, and within a day or two of the surgery, Lillie had recovered enough to be interested in her surroundings. Things were slow—scheduled patients weren't making it to the hospital because of the weather. Nurses found themselves with free time. Lillie talked with her nurse, Gail, about her own desire to be a nurse and Gail asked Lillie if she wanted to look around the hospital. "Sure," she said, feeling well enough to be a little bored.

The nurse took her in a wheelchair down to the first floor, and into the rotunda. It was evening and the lights around the rotunda bathed the statue in an ethereal pale yellow glow. This was the first time Lillie had seen The Divine Healer. Her first reaction was amazement at its size—she was sure the figure was thirty feet high. (Years later, when someone told her it was only ten feet tall, she was astonished.) She was a religious girl—on Sundays, she and her mother both sang in their own Methodist church and many other churches in the area, in a variety of services. She had been confirmed a few weeks before the appendicitis struck, and was feeling particularly religious, imbued with spirituality. Sitting in her wheelchair at the foot of the statue, she felt the radiance that many describe upon meeting *Christus Consolator*. She wanted to reach out and touch Him—but she held back, afraid it was forbidden. Even though marble is always cold, she had the sense that this marble would be warm. The statue gave her a sense of confidence, not just for herself but for all the other patients too. She knew that this was the front entrance of the hospital, and she felt that Jesus was standing there, blessing the health care providers as they went about their work of the day, thanking them as they left. *Jesus approves of what's being done in this hospital,* she thought, and she further narrowed her own personal goals, deciding that Hopkins was where she wanted to study nursing.

Unfortunately, five years later when Lillie was ready for nursing school, Hopkins had discontinued (temporarily) its nursing education program. So Lillie got her RN degree from Easton Memorial Hospital, closer to home, then married and moved to the West Coast for a couple of years. The marriage didn't work out, and Lillie moved back to Maryland, taking a succession of nursing jobs in several different Baltimore hospitals. She was a head nurse at Kernan

Hospital when Al Shockney came in as a patient. This honest, sincere, caring truck driver who managed to be sweet and gruff at the same time was the man for her, Lillie realized before long. They married in 1978, and two years later their daughter Laura was born. The birth was not without complications—Lillie needed an emergency cesarean section and had an allergic reaction to the anesthesia. "Nobody likes to put me to sleep," she says of the surgeries she has faced in her life.

She finally realized her goal of being a Hopkins nurse shortly after Laura was born, when she came to work as clinical nurse specialist for neurosurgeon George Allen. Allen's patients were among the most challenging a doctor can see—people with malignant brain tumors or fragile cerebral aneurysms resulting in life-threatening hemorrhages. The operations were long, often lasting more than six hours, and the hospital had not yet created the position of patient representative to keep waiting families informed of the patient's status as surgery progresses. Lillie often filled that role, reporting from the operating room to anxious relatives. She had a knack for soothing and reassuring, and her own warmth added comfort as she explained the details of what was going on in the operating room. But these were difficult cases, and sometimes comfort was needed from another source. Lillie often accompanied family members to the hospital rotunda to introduce them to The Divine Healer. (By that time, the Wolfe Street entrance had become the main lobby, and many patients passed through Hopkins without ever seeing the statue.) Lillie was glad she could do this. Sometimes she stayed with the people; others wanted to be left alone. The women, she observed, often wept when they first saw the statue.

When Dr. Allen left Hopkins, Lillie turned from clinical to administrative nursing. It was time to take a step back from hands-on care, she felt, and apply her experience and expertise at a broader level. By then she had earned her bachelor's degree in healthcare administration and was working on a master's in administrative science, which she received in 1988 from Johns Hopkins University. That was also the year she became director of performance improvement and utilization management for the entire hospital—a weighty title for a critical job. As managed care became firmly entrenched and cost containment an important consideration for everyone in healthcare, hospitals were setting up mechanisms to keep track of quality of care institution-wide. Lillie would be coordinating that effort.

It was a demanding job. Lillie was confronted with conflict every day. The hospital was asking doctors to do more and more, particularly in terms of documentation and medical record-keeping. Nurses had less time for patient care. Length of hospitalization was shrinking as insurers put a cap on what they would pay for and studies revealed that patients usually did just as well with shorter stays. Lillie was putting out fires every time she turned around. She worked long draining hours. "Put it away, Lil, you're going to burn out before you're forty," Al would tell her when she came home from work. But it wasn't until she had to confront problems with her own health that she really let herself step back.

The first scare came when she was only thirty-four. She felt a lump in her right breast. *Oh, dear Lord, I'm a young mother, please let this be nothing,* Lillie prayed. She looked at herself in the bathroom mirror, blue eyes, sandy hair, freckles, and thought, *If something serious was wrong, I would look different.* Still, she was afraid that she was going to lose her breast. Al was afraid he was going to lose *her.* But it turned out it *was* nothing—a blocked milk duct that disappeared with hot compresses. She gave heartfelt thanks for the good news: *God, thank You for Your kindness in sparing me. Thank You for allowing this experience to get me closer with Al, to let me know not to take my good health for granted.* Later Lillie and Al would wryly remember the episode as a dress rehearsal—the agonizing realization that something was there that shouldn't be, the pain as her breast was squished like a pancake for the mammogram, the anxious weekend of waiting for the results.

Four years later, in 1992, Lillie felt a similar lump in almost the same location. She was sure it was another blocked duct. There was some pain this time, but she tried compresses for a couple of weeks before she mentioned it to her doctor. Better get a mammogram, he told her, and for Lillie that meant walking from one part of the hospital to another. She hoped that the prompt attention and comprehensive service she got didn't have anything to do with her position at the hospital—she always felt she was being treated like a VIP and didn't like it. She hoped the general public got the same treatment. Feeling calm, she sat down later in the day to look over the mammograms with the radiologist. Yes, it did look like another cyst causing another painful blockage in the right breast, he told her. But he was also concerned about some spots he saw in the left breast, some "microcalcifications." They hadn't been evident on her last mammogram.

Many women learn from a mammogram that they have microcalcifications, microscopic calcium deposits that are benign 80 percent of the time. But they can be malignant or premalignant. They can appear as a single speck or a cluster. Sometimes calcifications indicate nothing more than a need for close monitoring, to see if they change from one mammogram to the next. But often biopsy is recommended.

Lillie's calcifications formed a horseshoe in the lower inner quadrant of her left breast. With her history, no one was taking any chances. Both her radiologist and gynecologist recommended that she see a breast surgeon and have the area biopsied. In the next couple of days, Lillie managed to shut down her emotions and apply her professional skills and the resources of her position to make a decision about a surgeon. She asked some nurses she trusted for their recommendations, and then studied the quality assurance data generated by her own office to determine who had experience with this procedure, who had the shortest length of stay for their patients, who had the fewest complaints filed about them. She decided on Charlie Yeo, a professor of surgery and oncology. Yeo had been at Hopkins more than twenty years, back to his medical school days, and his patients loved him. When Lillie called him, he saw her within days and told her he could do the biopsy later that week.

She had the open surgical biopsy performed at the Outpatient Center where, of course, everyone knew her. The procedure started with a mammogram, during which wires and dye were injected into her breast to identify the area for biopsy. It hurt so much, with her breast smashed in the vise-grip of the mammography machine, that she passed out. Finally that was done, and Al waited with her, holding her hand and squeezing reassurance, for the few minutes until Yeo called her into surgery. After injecting local anesthetic, he drained the cyst in Lillie's right breast, which only took seconds. In the left breast, making his way to the blue dyed area, he encountered another half-dozen cysts, which he drained. The tissue he took out was gray, and there was a lot of it. Charlie Yeo knew it didn't look good. "You have a diseased breast," he told Lillie, but it would be up to the lab to determine if it was cancer.

Yeo was leaving the next day for a five-day conference, and he wanted to be the one to tell Lillie her diagnosis. The wait was agonizing for her. The serenity prayer had always been very soothing to her and she found herself chanting it, almost like a mantra. *God, grant me the serenity to accept the things I cannot change, courage to change the things I can, and the wisdom to know the difference.* Without a definite diagnosis, she had told only her closest coworkers and family what was going on. Charmayne called several times a day from the Shore, anxious and unsettled, knowing that her own attitude wasn't doing anything to help Lillie, but unable to contain her fears. Lillie was back at work after two days, nursing a breast that was much more sore than she had expected. When she looked at it in the shower she couldn't believe the size of the indentation and incision, almost four inches long.

In her office the following Tuesday evening, the day before Yeo was due back, Lillie could no longer suppress her need to find out her diagnosis. She knew that the pathology report had been filed by then. She had access to all the hospital's databanks, and the information was only a few keystrokes away. *It's not going to be bad news,* she reassured herself. *It was just calcification, just more of these benign lumps that I get. It'll be fine.* She entered the pathology department's database and within a minute had her own report on her screen.

The words swam in front of her eyes, but one jumped out: "carcinoma." She saw it again, blinked, brought a couple more words into focus: "multiple foci," "intraductal carcinoma," "involving a . . . margin." More than a layperson, she knew what the words meant, couldn't keep the implications from flashing through her mind. "Multiple foci" meant that there was more than one section of her breast involved. The reference to the margin meant that there was almost definitely cancer tissue remaining in her breast. She put down the report, logged off the computer, stared at the blank screen, and expected the grim reaper to rise up off it. Thankfully, she was not alone—her secretary was in the office with her that evening, reminding her that breast cancer is not a death sentence, that hundreds of thousands of women live many years after diagnosis with this disease.

As Lillie left the hospital, she walked past the corridor to the Oncology Building and hurried by, almost running, with a dire, irrational feeling that the corridor was going to suck her in. She was headed for the Broadway entrance, the quickest way to get to her car that night, but she couldn't bear to look at the Christ statue as she came around the staircase and into the rotunda. She turned her head away. *I can't look at Him,* she thought. *I feel too scared. I've got to figure out what's wrong with me, how bad this is. I don't have enough information to know what I want to pray for.* She hurried past, and if someone had told her that His head turned to watch her, she would have believed it.

Thanks

Breasts are a strong part of any woman's identity. They help define her—physically, sexually, maternally. A large part of Lillie's self-image was tied up in her breasts. They were big—bra size 44D. She was fine with that. Since she'd been a teenager, they had preceded her into her every encounter with life, stalwart and proud. They'd gotten her through adolescence, dating, romance, one bad marriage, and now one very good one. She couldn't imagine that she'd be the same person without one of her breasts. Suppose she had a mastectomy and Al was repulsed by her body? Suppose she couldn't stand to be with herself in the shower? Suppose the cancer in her breast was already out in her body, already on its way to killing her?

In the United States, 180,000 new cases of breast cancer are diagnosed each year. One of every eight women will develop the disease—odds that have increased in recent decades. Women are living longer and breast cancer is discussed more openly than it was years ago. Public education, screening, and diagnosis are also much more aggressive. A generation ago breast cancer was a disease rarely spoken of directly. It was shameful to speak of something so private. Women died because they ignored symptoms in a part of their body that was not talked of except in the most intimate circumstances.

From the time she knew she had breast cancer, Lillie decided she would be open about her diagnosis and treatment. Many would feel the effects of her news. Working in a hospital and research center as she did, at least her coworkers would be somewhat knowledgeable. It might be harder with Laura, her daughter, now a vulnerable adolescent and experiencing new thinking of her own centered around her breasts. Charmayne and Frank were devastated—*Let me be the one who gets it, I'm older, I've lived my life,* Charmayne prayed in anguish. Al's reaction, from the beginning, back even to the first scare four years earlier, was consistent and solid, loving and supportive. He was a rock and always seemed to know the right reaction to Lillie's anxieties, whether it was a hug or a trip to the mall or a night of passion.

The night when Lillie read about her own "ductal carcinoma" in the computer, Al didn't come home from work until late. She had been wondering how she would tell him, knew she wouldn't call him while he was on the road and hit him with the frightening news when he still had hours of driving ahead of him. What would be the best words to use? Lillie, who always couched everything in a joke, couldn't think of a way to wrap anything funny around this. "I have breast cancer," she blurted out when Al walked through the door.

He stopped in his tracks, stunned, then asked the question that mattered most to him. "Are you okay?"

"Yes," she said. "Yes, I am."

He hugged her so tight she thought he was trying to squeeze the cancer out of her. "I've had four more years to love you since we had our first scare," he said. "We'll fight this together."

Al was more frightened than he let Lillie see. He didn't think of himself as much of a praying man. When a problem came up, his instinct wasn't to fall to his knees and ask God for help. Rather, he would say to himself, *What can I do to fix this?* Then later, when whatever it was got fixed, he'd utter a brief, *Thank You, God.* That night, though, before crawling into bed with Lillie and holding her all night long, he hung on to the bathroom sink and prayed as hard as he ever had in his life. *God, I know I don't say much to You, You don't see me that often. But, look, I really need something now. If You can help me and Lil this one time, I won't ask You again.*

~

Lillie had some decisions to make, but the course was pretty clear. Because there was more than one malignant site in her breast, she felt safest with a mastectomy, a surgical removal of the entire breast. Dr. Yeo confirmed that a mastectomy gave her the best chance for long-term survival. She set the date for July 14, 1992, several weeks away. She gave herself the extra time before surgery so she could clear her desk at work as much as possible.

Lillie was no stranger to mastectomy. She'd worked in the recovery room, seen women in the early 1970s wake up from a biopsy to find their breast removed. Growing up, she had been aware that two of her mother's friends were breast cancer survivors who had had mastectomies as relatively young women and gone on to live long and healthy lives. Miss Bertha and Miss Lena had been more guarded about their condition than women in the nineties. But Lillie was friendly enough with them so that she had heard the stories about losing a breast prosthesis in the swimming pool or having an inflatable bra pop in the pressurized cabin of an airplane. Her own sense of humor couldn't be kept down long, especially when twelve-year-old Laura asked questions like would Lillie's remaining breast be moved to the middle of her chest for balance, and could she bring the amputated breast home with her and keep it in a jar? Even as she began to tell her coworkers and a widening group of friends and colleagues throughout the hospital about her condition, she was making people smile with her. She sent Charlie Yeo a riddle cartoon she had drawn, two stick figures on either side of a big circle with a small circle in the middle of it, their hands guiding it. *"What's this a picture of?" "It's two men walking 'abreast.'"* Smiles and tears, they often came together. And flowers too—soon Lillie's office was filled with an outpouring of floral support from the many people who had come to admire and love her in her years at Hopkins.

While she waited for surgery, Lillie heard of several women who scheduled mammograms because of her experience. It was grim satisfaction, but satisfaction nonetheless, that her own misfortune might be saving someone else's life. In her prayers, she never asked "why me?" but she did want to find meaning from this horrible experience. *Dear God, let me live, let me survive this medical experience,* she prayed. *I know I have more responsibilities and duties to be fulfilled on this earth.*

Many women who have mastectomies have reconstruction at the same time, so that they never know the feeling of not having a breast. The two most common types of reconstruction done today are implants and the increasingly popular TRAM-flap procedure, in which a section of the patient's belly is moved and fashioned into a breast. But Lillie decided against reconstruction. It didn't seem right for her. Because she was so large-breasted, it would be difficult to approximate her remaining breast with an implant. And because of her troubles with anesthesia, the TRAM-flap operation, which could last ten hours or longer, seemed ill-advised.

The mastectomy without reconstruction is a relatively simple surgical procedure that takes a couple of hours and usually requires one night's hospitalization or less. (Many women now have mastectomies on an outpatient basis and go home the same day as surgery.) Lillie's surgery was scheduled for early morning, and Al dropped her off at the Hopkins Wolfe Street entrance, then went to park the car. Walking alone through the predawn hush in the dim corridors, Lillie was surprised to see longtime Hopkins chaplain Clyde Shallenberger walking down the hall toward her. He was a good friend. "What are you doing here at this ungodly hour?" Lillie asked him as they hugged. "There are no ungodly hours," he reassured her. "God is with us all the time."

In the past when she'd had anesthesia, Lillie had been bothered by the unpleasant hallucinatory jangle of an out-of-tune piano as she fell asleep. Going under for her mastectomy turned out to be a very different experience. Now, as she was drifting off, she heard her mother's clear powerful voice singing a hymn they both loved, *He Smiled On Me*. The familiar words gave her unexpected support:

> *Today on the highway I saw Him*
> *He gazed up and smiled at me*
> *Today on the highway I found Him*
> *Jesus of Galilee*
> *Oh, gentle and kind was His manner*
> *And though He made never a sound*
> *I felt as I gazed upon Him*

Thanks

That I stood in a presence divine.
Around Him the air it seemed hallowed
My soul felt the joy on His face
Around Him the earth reflected
The light of God's smile on His face.
The very same Jesus who suffered
The very same Jesus who trod
The valleys and banks of the Jordan
And His smile was the smile of God
Today on the highway I found Him,
He gazed up and smiled at me.

Charmayne, usually a diminutive powerhouse of stability and support for everyone else, was still having a hard time dealing with Lillie's illness. She had watched her own father die of prostate cancer,
and now she felt that she was watching her daughter in a similar battle and it didn't feel right; the natural order was disturbed. "I can't
stand it," she wept to Frank. "There is nothing fair about this. She
doesn't smoke or drink. All she is guilty of is working too hard."
Prayer helped, so Charmayne prayed, tearfully, for a miracle. She
contacted her own church and then other churches, far and wide, and
had Lillie put on their prayer lists. Lillie loved the idea that her name
was being spread through this spiritual network, and that her
mother's worries had led to something as constructive as prayer.

Lillie had gone out with Laura the week of the biopsy to buy
Laura's first bra. They managed to joke about the unfortunate timing, but Lillie's heart went out to her twelve-year-old. What a
crummy thing for a mother to do to a daughter at this tenuous stage
of life—suddenly, all anyone can talk about, and think about is
breasts! Laura tried to have a no-big-deal attitude but Lillie knew she
was holding in fear and confusion. Almost as soon as she woke up
from surgery in the recovery room and was moved to her own room,
Al presented her with a poem that Laura had written five days earlier:

<u>Appearance</u>
Nobody's perfect;
Just look at me
But if you really think about it
Who wants to be?

Beauty and glamour
Are nice to get
But it's what's inside that counts;
You must never forget.

I hope you understand
What I've been trying to say
I hope you get well soon
And I love you more and more each day.

Lillie felt overwhelmed by her daughter's simple wisdom and the fact that she had taken the trouble to express it in this way. In her brief twenty-four-hour hospitalization, Lillie also met with a volunteer from Reach for Recovery, a helping group for breast cancer survivors, with a particular emphasis on assisting with advice about fittings for a prosthesis and bra to hold it. Proper fitting for prostheses for women who have had mastectomies is a skillful art and science, and Lillie would go through a couple of steps before she was comfortable with the molded piece of silicone that would be her constant companion, except when she was sleeping or showering. She named her prosthesis Betty Boob.

Her plan was that Al wouldn't see her flattened chest, at least not in the foreseeable future. She would keep this slashed body part private between her and her doctor. But while she was still in the hospital, Al was in the room as Yeo removed the bandage, the surgeon casually asking Al to help so he would be able to change the dressings at home. Lillie was terrified that he would be repulsed by the incision. He was only matter-of-fact, though, wanting to help with the medical care. "It looks fine, we're going to be fine," he told Lillie. He was so relieved—this was still Lillie, with or without a breast didn't matter a whit to him.

During the mastectomy, some of Lillie's lymph nodes from her underarm were removed, to be dissected and examined for any traces of cancer cells. She was delighted when Dr. Yeo told her that the nodes were clear of cancer. Usually when cancer spreads from the organ where it originated out into the body, it follows a path through the nearest lymph nodes; thus if the lymph nodes are clear, chances are the cancer has not spread. The five-year survival rate for women with breast cancer that has not spread is a reassuring 97 percent. Lillie knew she still had to be concerned with her remaining breast and its tendency to develop cysts, but negative nodes were the closest thing to a clean bill of health that she could hope for.

She thanked God with a prayer she liked from an Eastern Orthodox Christian prayer book.

Loving God, Your healing power has saved me. You have sustained me in my weakness, supported me in my suffering, and set me on the road to recovery. By Your grace, I have found the strength to endure the hours of distress and pain. I have recovered, to express gratitude for all Your mercies by greater devotion to Your service. Blessed is the Lord, the Source of healing.

She slowly gained her strength back from surgery, eased her way back into work, started thinking life was almost normal. But "normal," Lillie soon began to think, meant continuing anxiety about her remaining breast. Six months after the mastectomy, a mammogram of the right breast showed a dense area that was slightly bigger than in the last mammogram. Another mammogram six months later showed another suspicious spot. A biopsy was scheduled for a year to the day from the mastectomy. Lillie and Al felt the familiar dread, but at least this time they knew what to expect. And this time, the news was good—the biopsy was negative. No cancer, just fibrosis.

A year later, though, in June 1994, another mammogram showed that the masses in her right breast had gotten bigger. A followup sonogram indicated that they were probably benign, but Dr. Yeo thought she should have another biopsy. Lillie had had enough. "I can't live like this," she wailed to Al, "I feel like I'm living from biopsy to biopsy. They're going to whittle this breast down a piece at a time."

In his clinical notes, Dr. Yeo wrote: "The patient has been incredibly concerned about her recent mammogram and was quite tearful during our conversation." He presented three options: do nothing but continue monitoring with mammograms, which he did not recommend; have the biopsy and proceed on the basis of that result; have a second mastectomy and forever banish the fear of breast cancer.

A preventive mastectomy is an extreme approach, but many high-risk women choose this option so they will not face year after year of worry and anxiety. Lillie knew this was what she wanted, even though this time she had trouble saying the word "mastectomy." Instead she spoke of "getting a roommate for Betty Boob."

Al was frightened. During one of his visits to Hopkins, he passed through the Broadway lobby and looked at the figure of Christ, his eyes drawn up to the serene face by a powerful force. He remembered saying two years ago that he was never going to ask God for anything again. *Jesus,* he prayed as he stood at the statue looking up, *I need Your help again.*

Lillie's right breast was removed on June 24, 1994. This time the postsurgical report showed that not only was there no cancer in the lymph nodes, there was none in the breast itself. There were, however, some "precancerous changes," and Lillie never regretted the operation. She was tremendously relieved that the breast was gone.

Now she could really move on. Before too long, she was joking with Al about the new stick-on nipples on the market, and what a great Christmas stocking-stuffer they would make.

Any woman who has had a breast removed worries about what it means for her sexuality. If she loses both of her breasts, like Lillie, not only does she have to worry about being attractive to her partner, but there is the added concern of whether the removal of two out of three of a woman's primary erogenous zones will stifle her own desire and enjoyment. Al made it his mission to convince Lillie that if you lose sensation in one place, it will intensify in another, and he went to work to prove it. Five weeks after the second mastectomy, he took Lillie on a vacation in the Poconos and showed her that sex could still be great.

Breast cancer had made Al and Lillie's marriage stronger in every way—emotionally, physically, mentally, sexually, spiritually. Lillie also found that her own experiences could be of benefit to other women facing the same ordeal. She started attending a support group and became involved as a volunteer counselor for other women. It made her long hours at the hospital even longer, but Al could always tell when she came home late if she'd been doing volunteer work because of the look of satisfaction on her face. It was time to seek that kind of satisfaction full time. She'd been doing the quality assurance work for ten years—well beyond the burnout period for most people in her position.

When the job of director of education and outreach for the Breast Center was posted, Lillie knew this was what she wanted to do. It was patient-focused work, not under the authority of a single department but encompassing the different disciplines that are involved with breast disease: radiology, surgery, oncology. Today the Breast Center is closely tuned to the opinions and advice of a corps of survivor volunteers who report to Lillie, and she has become a much-in-demand public speaker with engagements all over the country. Often she speaks of the role of humor in confronting breast cancer, with funny anecdotes about Betty Boob and her "roommate" Bobbie Sue.

In 1997 she published a book about her experience—*Breast Cancer Survivor's Club: A Nurse's Experience.*

Because of the disease she has now put behind her, she is able to empathize with suffering and pain and death. She is close to women who are much less fortunate than she was. Their stories are sometimes heartbreaking: young women with advanced breast disease, living only months after diagnosis and leaving young children behind; women who are rejected by their husbands when they get breast cancer; even women who lose their jobs because of breast cancer. For each, Lillie has practical and emotional support, advice, and prayer.

In her book, she wrote of how her work helped her make sense of her disease:

> *There is little doubt in my mind that I was meant to get breast cancer. It is rare that we learn while here on this earth why bad things happen to us. But I was blessed with being given the answer early on. It is so I can provide support to other club members who follow behind me. It also is so I can effect change in traditional treatment and think "out of the box" to develop ways that breast cancer treatment will be easier for women diagnosed in the future.*

Prayer remains a big part of Lillie's approach to this and any other issue in her life. She wants to put together an experimental study to investigate whether women who are the recipients of distant prayer, but don't know they are being prayed for, do better than women who are not prayed for. It is one of the most intriguing questions in the context of faith and healing.

And often, as she goes through the hospital, Lillie will stop at the foot of The Divine Healer and ask for help for the difficult cases she sees, and help for herself as she holds the hands of women in need.

> *For health of body and spirit, I thank You. Lord, I was broken and now I am whole; weary, but now am rested; anxious, but now*

Thanks

am reassured. I thank You for those who helped me in my need, who heartened me in my fear and who visited me in my loneliness. For the strength You gave me, O God, I give thanks to You. Blessed is the Lord, the Source of healing.

—LILLIE'S PERSONAL PRAYER

JAMES LANGE

Jimmy's Brain

*Dear Lord. This is Jim. I was wondering if
You could ask all my Guardian Angels to pray for
me to make my spells go away so I won't have to
have a hemispherectomy. Hope You are happy in
heaven.*

—JULY 17, 1998

Jimmy Lange's seizures began when he was seven, but his neurological problems dated back to the day of his birth—or even before. He had suffered a stroke, a rare complication in newborns, but in Jimmy's case the damage seemed to be minimal. He had mild cerebral palsy, the main symptom a slight paralysis on one side of his body (hemiparesis), which as he grew affected his speech, his gait, and the fine motor activities of his right hand. Jeff and Roree, his parents, were able to correct his walking problems with a brace on his right leg, and his slight handicaps had little effect on his daily life.

Jimmy had plenty of friends in his home town of Derry, New Hampshire, and his interaction with them and his three older siblings was full of the roughhousing, teasing, and competition common in any home. He was the baby of the family, and although his sister, April, and his brothers, Jeff and Rob, adored Jimmy and could be protective of him, they treated him like a normal boy—which by virtually all measures he was.

Jimmy did well academically, easily keeping up with his classmates. Although his fine motor skills were somewhat deficient—he could not tie his shoes and never mastered riding a bike—he took karate lessons, learned to swim, and even played basketball. Dribbling the ball was a problem—his opponents had little trouble stealing it from him—but he vowed he would not "retire" until he had scored a basket in a real game. He accomplished that goal when he was nine, to the cheers of the crowd, including his parents, in the stands. He was a thin, gangly boy with short brown hair, blue eyes, a huge smile, and an infectious optimism and endearing lack of self-pity. Nobody felt sorry for him since he did not seem to feel sorry for himself. During his early years, and even after the serious troubles began, there was nothing to indicate that this appealing, huggable little boy would come to a point where only prayer and the miracles of modern medicine could save him.

His parents weren't around to see Jimmy's first seizure, but his brothers and sister were. They saw their seven-year-old brother suddenly stand rigid, as though playing freeze tag, unable to move, a look of frightened bewilderment in his eyes. The rigidity didn't last for more than a few seconds, Jimmy was soon able to move again, and the incident might have been forgotten had it not happened again, then again, then again and again, often in more powerful and terrifying ways.

Sometimes Jimmy would talk right through the seizures. "I'm having one," he'd say to Roree as they stood in the kitchen, and she would tell him everything would be all right. But sometimes the seizures were more serious. Jimmy's body would tremble; his arms would twitch; his face would become blank, as though he were completely unaware of his surroundings. Often he would fall down, and there was no way for Roree or Jeff to hide their terror, or for Jimmy to hide his.

Soon, the entire family was held captive by Jimmy's epilepsy. Jeff worked for Home Depot, Roree sold advertising from their home, and together they ran a beach club on Beaver Lake in Derry. They lived in a sprawling, hundred-year-old house on the lake which they added to as the children came and grew and needed privacy. It was a good life, put together with hard work and dedication and love of each other and of God. But things took an unexpected turn when they entered what Roree called the EEG world, the focus of their lives fixated on the hectic activity in Jimmy's brain.

⁓

Within two weeks of Jimmy's first seizure, three more episodes occurred. Roree described them to the doctors at the local clinic who referred her to a neurologist in nearby Manchester. He ran a series of neurological tests and prescribed antiseizure medicines, but instead of improving, the seizures became longer and more violent. The doctor admitted he was baffled and referred the Langes to a pediatric neurology team at Boston Children's Hospital, an hour's drive from Derry.

Electroencephalograms taken there, even during one of Jimmy's seizures, showed no abnormal electrical activity, indicating a problem so deep within the brain that an EEG could not evaluate it. The neurologists could tell the Langes what was happening—as if they couldn't see for themselves—but were no closer to determining a cause. Jeff and Roree knew Jimmy was in expert hands at Boston Children's, but they were frustrated by the lack of answers—and their panic grew.

Jimmy started taking different drugs and then, as single drugs seemed to have little effect, drugs in combinations. Klonopin and Tegretol, Dilantin and Depakote and Frissium (which they had to get in Canada, because it was not FDA-approved); at one point, Jimmy was taking five drugs at a time. Each new regimen would bring momentary hope, and sometimes the seizures would stop for a few days. But always they would return with what seemed to be redoubled force.

Thanks

The Langes tried Jimmy on a ketogenic diet. High in fat, low in protein, and nearly carbohydrate free, the diet has been used to treat seizures since the 1920s and is still sometimes used on children who don't respond to more standard medications. It is an extreme remedy, beginning with two days of fasting at the hospital under close medical supervision, but the several theories as to why it works were irrelevant as far as Jimmy was concerned. After he had stayed five weeks on the diet, his seizures continued relentlessly.

Seizures are caused by electrical discharges in the brain that alter behavior, consciousness, or muscle tension. Doctors divide them into two main categories, partial or generalized. In a partial seizure, the excessive electrical discharge is confined to one section of the brain; a generalized seizure involves the whole brain. Partial seizures can be "simple," with the person experiencing odd or unusual sensations such as sensory distortions or the jerky movement of a body part; or "complex," in which consciousness is impaired and the sufferer feels dazed and confused and may wander around, mumbling purposelessly. Absence seizures (formally called *petit mal*) are generalized. The victim experiences a five- to fifteen-second loss of consciousness and has a dazed, disconnected affect. Tonic-clonic seizures (once called *grand mal*), also generalized, are the most severe. A person loses consciousness and becomes rigid (tonic phase), then begins twitching in the extremities (clonic phase). Severe injury can result from sudden falls or tongue-biting, and the spectacle is horrifying— even for doctors to see.

Jimmy experienced them all—partial and general, absence and tonic-clonic—with varying degrees of severity and frequency, "without warning and without mercy, at any time and any place," as Jeff wrote in the journal he began to keep some time later. One day Jimmy would have more than one hundred seizures, the next day "only" three. Any sudden physical action could bring one on—a stumble, an unexpected bump. Jimmy would go rigid, shake and fall over, his arms straight out. Sometimes he didn't remember what had happened. His bruises were a solemn reminder.

His brothers and sister tried to keep Jimmy's life as normal as possible, including him in their activities, treating the episodes with feigned casualness, and Jimmy tried to behave normally too. But as the seizures continued, he grew more and more afraid, more and more insular, clutching at a parent's or sibling's arm not because he was having a seizure but because he feared he was about to.

For months, as different regimens were tried and failed, the family remained optimistic. This medicine didn't work? No matter, the next one would. The next prescription, the next combination, the next *doctor* would provide the answer and the seizures would cease. In their different individual ways, Jeff and Roree turned to prayers. Both Christians, they were regular churchgoers, and both had an unshakable faith in God; each felt that He was walking with them and that there was, somehow, a reason for their trial.

> *In your day of trouble may the Lord be with you! May the God of*
> *Jacob keep you from all harm.*
> *May He send you aid.*
> *May He remember with pleasure the gifts you have given Him,*
> *your sacrifices and burnt offerings.*
> *May He grant you your heart's desire and fulfill all your plans.*
> *May there be shouts of joy when we hear the news of your victory,*
> *flags flying with praise to God for all that He had done for*
> *you.*
> *May He answer all your prayers.*
>
> —PSALMS 20:1–5

A strange sound, a cross between a gasp and a scream, came from the living room, where Jimmy was. In the kitchen, Roree dropped the plate she was holding and rushed to her son. He was lying on the couch, shaking all over, his skin a frightening shade of blue, his expression so filled with terror it almost broke her heart. He couldn't answer her questions, couldn't communicate at all. *He's never been this gone before,* Roree thought, and she dialed 911 with trembling fingers. It took four or five minutes for the attack to end, and by that time the medics were almost at the house. Jimmy was hospitalized overnight; his doctors speculated that this tonic-clonic seizure was a result of coming off a medication too quickly.

But then, incredibly, the seizures began to subside. For a while, they occurred only when Jimmy was sleeping; then they stopped altogether. The family held its collective breath. Days went by, then weeks and months. Nothing. Could the ordeal be over?

Fourteen seizure-free months passed. Jimmy continued taking Klonopin, which had seemed to help him most with the fewest side effects, but no one knew if the drug had stopped the seizures or if Jimmy had simply "outgrown" them. No matter; nobody changed the regimen. "We dared to hope," Jeff wrote in his journal. "Realistically hope."

But then, in the spring of 1997, when Jimmy had just turned ten and was in the fourth grade, the "spells" (as he called them) returned. This time they were more powerful, more frightening, more savage than ever before. And with no more explanation than when they had ceased.

Oh gosh, we're going through it again, Roree despaired. Jimmy's life deteriorated quickly. He fell many times a day. Danger lurked on a flight of stairs or a walk outside. Physical activity all but ceased; showers were forbidden; even as simple an act as standing might bring on an attack.

Becoming embarrassed by his condition and wanting to avoid social contact, Jimmy kept more and more to himself. His brothers and sister continued to encourage him to join them on outings, but he resisted. The only safe place was the floor, he argued. So he would lie for hours playing video games, wheedling Roree even to serve him his meals on the floor. She complied, because all she wanted was to make life easier for her son.

Autumn came, and a new school year, but Jimmy stayed home.

Jimmy's Brain

School was too perilous; Jeff and Roree arranged for a tutor. Just when a child's world should be expanding, Jimmy's was closing in around him, his home becoming a virtual cell.

It's no way for a boy to live. Please, God, give Jimmy a break, Roree prayed, taking some comfort from the act of praying itself but not knowing where to look for hope for her son. Medical consultations and different combinations of drugs started again. The Boston Children's neurologist gave them a book called *The Epilepsy Diet Treatment: An Introduction to the Ketogenic Diet* to explain the philosophy behind the diet. And he recommended another by the same author, *Seizures and Epilepsy in Childhood: A Guide for Parents*. The writer was John Freeman, pediatric neurologist and director of the Pediatric Epilepsy Center at The Johns Hopkins Hospital. In his books, Freeman described a procedure the Boston Children's doctors were now openly discussing—a hemispherectomy.

⁓

A hemispherectomy is exactly what the name implies: the removal of half the sphere of the brain. In Jimmy's case it would be the left side, since it had long been apparent that this was where the stroke at birth had caused serious damage, resulting in chaotic and overwhelming electrical impulses that caused the seizures. Was it possible that taking out half of Jimmy's brain would cure his seizures?

What a decision! It was a fearsome prospect, and Roree and Jeff anguished over it. What would Jimmy's life be like, assuming he survived the operation? Would he be able to think as well as he did now? Would he be able to run, play, use his hands, walk, *speak?* What if the cost of stopping the seizures was the end of a fulfilling life? What is the fate of an eleven-year-old boy with half a brain?

Without saying anything to Jimmy, Roree began researching hemispherectomies on the Internet, and learned that this rare operation had been performed more at Hopkins than anywhere else— eighty procedures compared to a handful at all other medical institutions in the United States combined. From what she read, the success rate seemed promising. Most of the children recovered from the hemispherectomy and remained mostly seizure free. Usually, there was some partial paralysis on the side of the body opposite the half of the brain that was removed. But in children, she learned, the brain is adaptive enough for the remaining hemisphere to take over most of the functions of the part that has been removed.

Roree reasoned that if the operation was to be performed at all, Hopkins would be the place, in consultation with Dr. Freeman. Yet still she hesitated, too frightened to begin taking steps to make it happen. Jeff was more positive. From the time he first learned of the possibility, he was open to the idea, believing that a problem as extreme as Jimmy's needed an extreme solution.

At last, before making a final decision, Roree decided to get more of a feel for Hopkins itself, to take in its emotional atmosphere and get a sense of the physical plant. In June 1998 she flew to Baltimore, rented a car, and drove to the city landmark. She parked in the garage adjacent to the hospital, and walked to the street and around the sprawl of Victorian brick buildings, her mind in turmoil. *Please, God,* she prayed, *give me a sign. If Jimmy is supposed to have a hemispherectomy, please give me a sign.*

In its 109 years of existence, Hopkins had grown from the original simple cluster of buildings to an architectural beehive, a succession of buildings linked through corridors, tunnels, and lobbies on the interior. It can be entered through doors on several different streets, and Roree used the one on Broadway, the hospital's original entry, which leads directly to the huge figure of Christ at the center of the rotunda. She stopped. Looked up. Saw the outstretched arms, the bent head. She truly believed God had led her to this spot. God's spirit was alive in this hospital and she felt it within her. *Oh, yes,* she thought. *This is the sign I was looking for. Jesus will take care of my son here.*

After further investigation, she flew back home and called Dr.

Freeman's office, expecting to get an answering machine or to be put on a waiting list for an opening months in the future. What she got instead was a long conversation with Diana Pillas, coordinator-counselor for the Epilepsy Center and John Freeman's right-hand person for more than twenty years; a half hour on the phone with Freeman himself; and an appointment in two days if she could gather together Jimmy's records in so short a time.

All this she reported to Jeff with an optimism he had not seen in her for four years. Yet both knew that the most important person had yet to be consulted: their son Jimmy.

Jimmy did not like the idea of a hemispherectomy. He felt like he was walking through a house of horrors, never knowing what was going to happen next, but knowing it was going to be scary. He was always tense, waiting for the next episode. But sometimes he wasn't even sure he wanted his seizures to end. Each seizure allowed the release of the continually building tension. Suppose after the operation the tension kept building with no release? That was a terrible thought. Life wasn't so frightening now that his parents let him stay on the floor most of the time, and he didn't have to go to school. Suppose he still had the seizures after they removed half his brain. Suppose he died! It seemed like a lot of bad supposes.

Still, he agreed to accompany his parents to Hopkins and at least *meet* with the new set of doctors who wanted to cut out half his brain. Before he saw them, though, he wrote the prayer which opens this chapter. Maybe his Guardian Angels would save him. Maybe the seizures would stop on their own, and he wouldn't have to be scared as he was now.

At Hopkins, he met Freeman, Diana Pillas, and Benjamin Carson, the pediatric neurosurgeon who would perform the actual operation. It seemed a good omen to everyone that Jimmy's T-shirt and Freeman's tie both pictured Tigger, the ebullient *Winnie the Pooh* character. It helped Jimmy concentrate on what Freeman had to say. What he said, Roree and Jeff thought, was expert, honest, and clear.

Roree had read about Ben Carson, one of the stars in the Hopkins constellation. Youthful looking and low key, he had gained international attention for some of the daring and demanding procedures he had performed—separating Siamese twins joined at the head, removing brain tumors other surgeons had refused to touch, intrauterine surgery on the brain of a fetus. Not only had he performed eighty hemispherectomies, he was also in great demand as a motivational speaker for young people, drawing on his own life as an example.

In adolescence, Carson had nearly killed a friend in what turned out to be a life-changing episode. When only a belt buckle saved the boy from Carson's knife, young Ben prayed for guidance to curb his anger. Later, he turned to medicine and in his books and his many speeches he spoke about the two major influences in his life: his mother and God. "There's no reason to be ashamed of God," he tells the young people he speaks to. "You do your best, and you let God do the rest."

The Langes liked what they heard. Roree and Jeff were impressed by the combination of advanced medicine and age-old spirituality Carson espoused, and they left Hopkins feeling that the hemispherectomy was Jimmy's best chance for a normal life.

They spent the summer trying to convince their son. But still he resisted. Frightened and unsure, he vacillated for weeks. Yes, he'd say one day, no, the next, until at last he agreed to be put on the surgery schedule and again visit Hopkins to talk more about it.

The operation was tentatively scheduled for October, but first Jimmy was given a Wada test (named after the Japanese neurologist who devised it), which evaluates how the brain will respond to a hemispherectomy. A short-acting anesthetic is injected into the brain through the carotid artery, one side at a time. With each half of the brain serially "asleep," the functions on each side—primarily speech, but also memory and motor performance—can be localized and assessed. In Jimmy's case, the results could not have been more encouraging. Speech, for example, was entirely localized to the undamaged right half of his brain. It seemed that the procedure had a good chance of causing minimal problems to that essential function.

Because the chaotic electrical signals were coming from Jimmy's left hemisphere, it also seemed the surgery would mean an end to the seizures. But Carson and Freeman could not guarantee it, and Jimmy wanted guarantees. The final decision about surgery was his, and it was his parents' wishes, not his own belief, that had allowed him to come even this far. He wanted to feel the way they did, but he couldn't. He prayed for another answer, prayed that the seizures would go away. *Please, God, why can't all this just be done with?* He kept the extent of his doubts to himself, but the day before the scheduled surgery, in a meeting with his parents, Freeman, Diana Pillas, and a neurology resident, Jimmy turned to Freeman and said, "I don't know why we're talking like this. I'm not going to have the surgery."

Roree and Jeff gasped. *This isn't happening,* thought Roree, who by now had put all her faith in the surgery. *God, I don't know if I can go back to that world of listening in terror for every sound. For seizures being part of every day, every hour.*

"That's fine," she heard Freeman say quickly. "We won't operate if you don't want us to." He paused and stared into Jimmy's eyes. "But you can't stay the way you are. This isn't a life. You're too bright. You can't stay out of school. You cannot spend your life on the floor."

Jimmy was upset and returned to the waiting room, where he joined his brothers and sister. They talked to him gently, but with emotion. They were all in favor of the hemispherectomy. As he listened to their urgings, he felt their love and support gave him the strength to finally make the decision. They would be there for him, no matter what. He agreed to the operation.

Thanks

That night, October 5, the family paid a visit to the Jesus statue and wrote down their prayers:

Dear Lord Jesus,
When they operate on my son tomorrow, please keep Your angels close.
                                                              Roree

Keep James under Your protective wing and help guide the hands of those who will be performing the operation.
                                                              Dad

Dear Lord Jesus
Please guide the surgeon's hands and keep a watchful eye on James as he is operated on today. Please give him comfort today and the many days of recovery to come.
                                                 Aunt Deb and family

On days when he's operating, Ben Carson is usually at the hospital by seven A.M. Preparations for surgery include reviewing CAT scans, running the procedure through in his head—and praying. Praying is as much a part of surgery for Carson as washing his hands. Since he came to Hopkins as an intern twenty-one years ago and first saw the statue of Jesus in the rotunda, he has felt a deep satisfaction at the hospital's acknowledgment of a higher power. He prays for all his patients, asks them to pray, and prays *with* patients who request it. "I have no doubt prayer works," he says.

April, Jeff, Jr., and Rob were at Hopkins with their parents, aunt, and grandparents for Jimmy's surgery. As he waited with them all before going into the OR, Jimmy proposed an alternative. "Just give me a knife and an ice cream scoop and I'll do it myself." He grinned. "Of course, I'll need some Play-Doh to fill up the hole."

Now that he had decided on this course, he had no second thoughts. But Jeff, walking with him into the OR, felt the enormity of it all hit him hard, the cold tile floors and stainless steel doors like a giant freezer in which the rest of his son's life would be decided. He tried not to communicate his dread. "Dad, I'll take over from here," Jimmy murmured as Jeff helped him up onto the operating table.

In the waiting room down the hall, his family provided Jeff the human warmth to ward off the chill of the OR. They captured a corner to wait out the day, comforting and supporting each other and praying for Jimmy as the hours went by.

Prayers were said for Jimmy from both near and far. A prayer chain had been organized by friends at Derry Christian School. People were signed up to pray at fifteen-minute intervals from seven-thirty A.M. to nine-thirty P.M., the expected duration of the operation and recovery room time. It wasn't only a family, but an entire community helping Jimmy with the procedure. In those grueling hours, Roree felt too numb to pray herself and gained comfort by collecting the prayers of others. More than 250 cards and prayers had arrived from friends at home and well-wishers who had heard about Jimmy through a local newspaper article.

On one card, there was a handwritten cross, crayon-drawn flower, and short message: *Jesus knows you, loves you and cares deeply for you.* And on the front of the card, this letter:

Dear Jimmy, I read about your illness and situation in the news-paper. I want you to know how much we all care, but especially how much the Greatest Physician loves and cares for you—Jesus. Our prayer is for His healing power to touch your lives—physical, emotional, psychological, spiritual. May He comfort you through-out this time, may He give the doctors wisdom and skill in their

Thanks

*treatment of you both, may you know the peace and love of God
now and always. In Jesus' name, I pray these things for you.*

Love, Deborah

Ben Carson says a brief prayer at the beginning of each operation: *God, give me wisdom and guidance.* Vivaldi plays through the sound system. For this and any hemispherectomy, there are teams of people in the operating room: Carson, a neurosurgery resident who will assist him, the scrub nurse and circulating nurse, the anesthesiology team, a neurology team, and in Jimmy's case John Freeman himself, who spent some time watching the procedure.

At seven A.M., the anesthesia began running into the IV line in Jimmy's arm, and he was unconscious in seconds. It was no ice cream scoop Carson and his associates used to take out half of Jimmy's brain, but an array of fine-edged precision tools. The procedure involves hours of meticulous, exacting, and incremental excisions, and the goal is to remove the tissue with as little blood loss and vessel damage as possible.

Jimmy's head had already been shaved, and the first step was to get to his brain. A first incision into the scalp was followed by a thin trickle of blood. The head, draped in green cloth and set off from the body by the sheaths of surgery, didn't seem attached to a boy any more. It had become a surgical field, distinct and contained, and for the next eight hours would be the intense focus of the outer edge of medical technology.

Soft-spoken and unfailingly polite, Carson often explains what he's doing as he goes along. "Make one definitive incision, rather than stop and start," he instructed as he cut Jimmy's scalp into four quadrants. With these incisions, blood began to flow copiously, and Carson and Tushar Goradia, the neurosurgery resident, were kept busy cauterizing blood vessels and mopping with sponges as they peeled back the scalp sections and secured them with clamps.

The skull is a thick, unyielding bone, resistant to intrusion. It takes several steps to open. Carson drew a series of dots around the circumference of Jimmy's skull, and he and Goradia then drilled a burr hole into each dot. They scraped out the holes with a curette, enlarging them, then sawed between the holes with a craniotome, a small circular saw with a rapidly rotating blade specifically designed to cut the skull. "Before you start prying up, go to every hole and loosen everything that can be loosened," Carson advised, and the surgeons gently pried the sections apart with spatulas, and finally lifted the skull to reveal the dura, the tough membrane that covers the brain.

Carson used surgical scissors to cut the dura in a C-shape, and then down the middle of the C to split it in two sections to be rolled back and clipped. Nearly an hour after the surgery began, the brain was visible. To the professional eyes of Carson and his team, the stroke damage to Jimmy's left brain was clearly visible, though a layman would see only what looked like a mass of fat bloody worms.

The actual removal of the brain was done in sections, moving from lobe to lobe with forceps and scissors and spatulas, millimeter by painstaking millimeter, with cotton pads inserted for temporary spacing and constant cauterization and sponging to stem the blood flow. As pieces of Jimmy's brain were removed, they were labeled and dropped into preservative trays, for analysis later in the lab. Carson describes this part of the operation as "grunt work." But the need for precision and caution never lessens. "I can't overemphasize," he tells his associates, "be careful. It may look like things are going nicely, but as soon as you get cavalier and start tugging, it'll mean trouble."

For five grueling hours, the surgeons cut away the damaged left hemisphere of Jimmy's brain. While the removal of such a large amount of tissue would leave Jimmy's head a little lopsided through the recovery period, eventually the cavity would fill with cerebrospinal fluid to offset the missing material.

Thanks

Hourly reports from the hospital patient representative eased the simmering tension in the waiting room. The reports were consistent: things were going smoothly; there was no need for concern. Still, question after question ran through Jeff's mind. *What's happening now in the OR? What's happening to Jimmy?* With all his anxiety, he nevertheless experienced a feeling of peace. The day was in the hands of Ben Carson—and God. Everything would be okay. He began keeping the journal that would detail his son's journey back from surgery.

It was not until surgery was ending at around six P.M.—the dura stitched back together, the skull reattached with titanium plates and screws, the scalp stapled closed—that there was the first and only bit of trouble in the OR. Jimmy's blood pressure started to drop precipitously, and when the operation was complete he was rushed to the CAT scanner. The scan revealed no apparent problem, and transfusing more blood brought the pressure back up.

Jimmy's family saw him for a brief moment when he was transported to the CAT scan. His head was wrapped in bandages, only a small circle of his face visible, and he seemed to be asleep. But an hour later, coming back from the scan, he was awake. Before the operation Roree and Jimmy had made a deal: when he woke up from surgery and knew who he was, knew he was all there, he would flash his mother a thumbs-up sign. "Mom, he has something to give you," a nurse said to Roree as Jimmy was wheeled into the recovery room. Roree looked down at her son who weakly but surely lifted his thumb toward the heavens. At that moment, she knew in her heart he had survived, he was going to make it.

An hour and a half later in the recovery room, Roree bent over her son and whispered, "Jim, you look great." Jimmy's voice was cracked and barely audible. "Don't lie to me, Mom."

A thumbs-up and a quip. Jeff and Roree knew that as battered as he might be, their little boy was still there. Now all they had to do was pray for a successful recovery.

Jimmy's Brain

Two days ago You, Lord, watched a doctor perform a miracle. Now my son lives with half a brain and is seizure free. Keep watch over him, Lord, as he heals—let all decisions be the best for him to heal.

Roree
October 8, 1998

For the first few days after the operation, Jimmy spent most of the time sleeping. By the end of the first week, he was spending longer periods awake and communicating more and more. At first, he was barely able to speak above a whisper in a voice that was squeaky and strained. But it quickly came back to normal. He responded automatically to simple questions:

"Are you hungry?"

"No."

"How do you feel?"

"Not so good."

He wished everyone would leave him alone and let him sleep. Consciousness sometimes was too much for him—the questions, the fatigue, the doctors and nurses and therapists who kept coming by.

Roree was inclined to coddle Jimmy, but Jeff pushed him toward rapid recovery. For Jimmy's father, every increment of progress was an emotional milestone. "Each time he makes a change that brings him closer to home, I feel peace come upon me," he wrote in his journal when Jimmy was able to talk normally. "There are so many times I find the tears at the edge of my eyes. Whether I'm looking right at him, hearing his voice, or just thinking about him. The whole situation can overwhelm you if you let it. My focus is always on looking down the road."

Nine days after the operation, the physical therapist got Jimmy on his feet. *My poor boy,* Roree thought, aching as she looked at him. Jimmy was shaky, leaning to his right, his mouth open, his eyes fixed. He took halting steps down the corridor, about thirty in all, leaning on the therapist, before she and Jeff finally let him get back in the chair. The next day Jeff and Roree took him outside in the wheelchair to the hospital courtyard where he could feel the cool October air on his face. Then they wheeled him to the Jesus statue, hoping for an animated reaction. But Jimmy remained quiet, listless, expressionless, interested only in getting back to bed.

Jeff and Roree alternated custodial duty, one spending the night in the hospital with Jimmy, the other sleeping at the Children's House, a facility for families of seriously ill patients. It became the Langes' home away from home. Rob flew down to visit on the weekend ten days after the surgery and by then Jimmy was demonstrating more and more signs of his old self. After one morning, Jeff wrote:

This is the best morning I've had so far. It started out with Jimmy waking up about 5, telling me he hasn't been able to sleep. I remind him that he's been asleep for the last 8 1/2 hours. It's true that he's awakened in the middle of the night, but Jimmy does most of the tasks they require in his sleep. We talk just a bit and the two of us continue to fade in and out of sleep.

Finally around 7:30 we make the effort to get our butts up. We make my bed, get him propped up in his, turn on the TV, brush our teeth, and give mom a call. We flip through the TV channels trying to find some cartoons. We finally find one called Louie . . . It's about a fat kid and he actually narrates the cartoon. About five minutes into the cartoon, there is a scene with three kids running down a path and Louie following them. Louie is not running, he's walking just as a short fat kid would be. This makes me laugh out loud and I turn to Jim to say, isn't that funny? Out of the corner of his mouth, the left side to be exact, comes this smile.

Jimmy's Brain

It's only half a smile, but it's the best thing that could ever have happened. Jim's sense of humor was returning and at this very moment my heart was being renewed with faith. I never questioned it. The moment would come. It lifted me right off the ground. These are the moments we thank the Lord. I continued to make him smile more and more. I couldn't wait for Roree to see her little boy smile at her.

~

Jimmy remained grudging with his smiles over the next few days, acting irritated at the constant quizzing to test his memory. Who are Rob's three best friends? What's your address? Where do your grandparents live? Who was your third-grade teacher? Jimmy answered, without hesitation and without error. Whatever the hemispherectomy had removed, it wasn't his memory. One residual effect for all children is impaired peripheral vision. Jimmy couldn't see sideways to the right, and it affected his walking and general equilibrium, as did the slight hemiparesis. The therapists taught him to turn his head and scan the periphery to compensate, first at Hopkins, and then at Mount Washington Children's Hospital in north Baltimore, where he was transferred for further rehabilitation two weeks after the surgery.

By then Jimmy was moving around, making jokes. Throwing punches at his dad when Jeff tried to motivate him from the reclining position he still favored. The Mount Washington regimen was "punishment," Jimmy declared. But he was walking on his own, his coordination more relaxed than before the operation. And he felt like he was thinking more clearly and quickly than ever before, maybe because his brain was no longer blunted by the antiseizure medications.

As he regained his energy, Jimmy focused on the reason he'd had the surgery in the first place. Were the seizures really gone? His parents were convinced they were—but they weren't the ones who'd experienced them in the first place. Jimmy's recovery was so swift that the projected four weeks at the rehab hospital were abbreviated to three, then two. Roree made a calendar, marking off the seizure-free days, one after another after another. One day, shortly before he would leave for home, Jimmy stood at the end of a long corridor at the hospital and looked down its length. Corridors had been his nemesis for so long—places to fear, places where seizures were bound to happen. He started walking and felt no fear. For the first time he felt his ordeal was over. He wasn't going to have another seizure, and he thanked God for it.

"I'm happy I don't have the seizures, and I'm happy I had the surgery," he told his parents in quiet triumph. "They found a cure for epilepsy, and I got it."

On the day Jimmy was discharged from the rehab hospital, he and Jeff drove the couple of miles downtown to Hopkins. They wanted to walk around and say good-bye. In the Broadway lobby, they stood together for a moment, looking up at the giant statue that seemed to have played such a pivotal role in the events of the past months. Then they wrote in the prayer book, first Jimmy, then Jeff.

Thank You, Lord, for letting the hemispherectomy work and getting rid of my seizures. Thank You for letting me go home to see my family.

Jimmy
October 29, 1998

Thank You, Lord, for giving the gift of life back. The four-year battle is over and life begins for Jimmy this day.

The Dad
October 29, 1998

AFTERWORD
Sacred Ground

$\mathbf{I}$n my years as a healthcare chaplain, I have always felt that interacting with individuals during the most vulnerable (and arguably the most intimate) moments of their lives, as they face their own mortality, is a supreme privilege—an invitation to walk with them through the sacred ground of their own souls. In this book, we have offered others a brief glimpse into the frequently undisclosed country of the spiritual life of a few patients and their families as they confronted serious, life-threatening illnesses while undergoing the best of what scientific medicine has to offer at The Johns Hopkins Hospital.

Coming face to face with death is something all human beings must do at least once. It is our hope that reading these stories will inspire others to look inward, and outward, to their own spiritual resources when that time comes for them, and to realize that such times are never faced alone if one's spiritual eyes are open.

Johns Hopkins, this hospital's namesake, was brought up in the Society of Friends, the Quaker religious tradition. Its early influence was a significant factor in his establishment of the hospital. The hallmark of spirituality in the Society of Friends is the affirmation of an individual's "Inner Light"—a spiritual central nervous system placed by God into every human being. This "Inner Light" from God is seen as having nothing to do with creeds or religious practices; instead, every human being is seen as a shrine and altar to God. Historically, Friends denied the validity of professional clergy, religious liturgy, or sacramental ministry. They held a profound respect for the dignity, worth, and equality of every man, woman, and child, since each held a spark of God's divine nature. With that understanding, it is no surprise that Friends tended to be exemplary in providing for human physical, social, and spiritual needs within society.

In Johns Hopkins' letter to the first board of trustees of the hospital on March 10, 1873, the Friends' influence can be clearly seen in the following excerpts:

> *The indigent sick of the city and its environs, without regard to sex, age, or color, who may require surgical or medical treatment . . . shall be received into the Hospital . . .*
>
> *It will be your highest duty to secure for the service of the Hospital surgeons and physicians of the highest character and greatest skill.*
>
> *I desire you to establish . . . a training school for . . . nurses . . . to care for the sick in the Hospital wards, and will enable you to benefit the whole community by supplying it with a class of trained and experienced nurses.*
>
> *. . . It is my especial request that the influence of religion shall be felt in and impressed upon the whole management of the Hospital; but I desire, nevertheless, that the administration of the charity shall be undisturbed by sectarian influence, discipline or control.*

At a time when all hospitals were administered by religious organizations, this call to uphold nonsectarian spiritual values was revolutionary (and given the current climate of a nonsectarian approach to spiritual care in the medical environment, downright prophetic).

Sacred Ground

In writing this afterword, I've been asked to highlight issues of spiritual care at The Johns Hopkins Hospital that have not been directly addressed in these stories of patients and their families. That is an awesome task to undertake within the constraints of a few pages. Let me begin with a discussion of what the stories you have just read did and did not tell you.

The literary device used to tie together the stories of this book is the contact of patients (and some physicians) with the hundred-year-old statue of Christ standing beneath the dome in the rotunda of The Johns Hopkins Hospital. And while the statue represents for some the compassion, love, and promise of divine healing inherent in all world religions, for others the statue may represent a sectarian Christian bias that runs counter to more modern sensibilities of religious and spiritual pluralism. The use of the statue as a literary thread, while enriching the context of the stories told here, does not express the fuller richness of the spiritual lives of many Hopkins patients and staff who come here from Jewish, Muslim, Hindu, Buddhist, Shinto, or other religious and spiritual backgrounds.

Spiritual care at Johns Hopkins embraces the fullness of religious and spiritual practices in a wide variety of ways, a few of which I will illustrate below. The stories in this book illuminate only a narrow band of this full spectrum—those for whom the statue of The Divine Healer was a fulcrum for the exercise of their spiritual faith.

These stories are ultimately *not* about miraculous healing, whether mediated by cutting-edge medical science, divine intervention, or some combination of both. These stories are instead about how one finds spiritual wholeness in the midst of the struggle with the reality of mortality—one's own or that of a loved one.

The word "wholeness" is actually a weak term for the Jewish idea embodied in the Hebrew word "shalom." "Shalom" carries connotations of completeness, soundness, welfare, and peace, and includes shades of healthy community with family, nation, the natural world, and God. Finding this "shalom" is the ultimate goal of all spiritual expressions.

Afterword

Isn't it ironic that for many this journey toward "shalom" either begins or finds its completion in moments bracketed by the specter of death?

Part of the ancient wisdom of religion's involvement in healing practices was the ability of the shaman (the physician/priest) as an emissary of God's healing power to provide not just the possibility of cure but also strength, hope, and meaning to life and death, even when cure was not possible. These stories celebrate the discovery of spiritual wholeness in the depths of human suffering.

To be sure, the human spirit soars when our prayers of healing for ourselves or our loved ones come true. But is the spirit no less enlightened or made less whole when we confront the imminent, and immanent, reality of death and find transcendent meaning in human life despite our finitude? These stories highlight both aspects of this equation, but the natural human bias present in these narratives emphasizes the hope of both wholeness and healing.

The stories shared in this book are focused, properly, on the human beings who walked through their own "shadow of the valley of death" and came out on the other side with a message of hope and inspiration for us all. These stories are about much more than the skill and compassion of doctors, nurses, social workers, technicians, food service workers, and housekeepers. Patients often take for granted the skill and compassion of healthcare workers, and their expectations may even be higher for staff in a world-renowned institution such as Hopkins. Most of these stories are *not* about the spiritual perspective of the staff at Hopkins—although the silent witness of their own spirituality and values can, and does, have a profound effect on patients' healing processes, and physicians are featured in two of the chapters. Nor are these stories about professional spiritual care or the hospital chaplain, who may or may not have been part of the process of healing and wholeness of the patients involved. They *are* about individual expressions of personal spirituality exhibited by patients or their loved ones during their health crises.

That said, in a book on spirituality, prayer, and healing, it would be a profound disservice to the subject, and my chosen profession, if I did not highlight some of the contemporary issues in spiritual care and health.

Religion, faith, and personal spirituality have had a role in the healing process since the beginning of recorded history. All the advances in rational, scientific medicine over the last century have not diminished the role of spirituality in the lives of patients one whit, if recent attention in the national media is any indication. In fact, new medical research has actually come full circle, showing that there may be scientific data that suggest significant correlations between personal faith and health.

The research into this nexus between spirituality and medicine is still relatively new, and not without some controversy. There are some who feel that such research is a step backward to a more primitive and superstitious understanding of health and healing. Others see spirituality as irrelevant to medical care as political orientation. Still others worry that this interest in spirituality is motivated by those with a religious dogma to proselytize. But there are also those who entered the healing arts with a sense of a divine vocation to alleviate the suffering of their fellow human beings. Their practice of medicine is infused with their own spiritual perspectives, even though they may never utter a word of it to their patients. And there are healthcare providers who see themselves as atheist or agnostic, but out of respect for their patients as whole persons, may elicit discussions of their patients' spiritual needs and resources to better understand and encourage all modalities that may foster healing.

While the full spectrum of thought and feeling about spirituality and medicine is present at Hopkins to varying degrees, it is instructive to note that Sir William Osler, the first physician in chief at Johns Hopkins before leaving to become Regis Professor of Medicine at

Oxford University, wrote an article entitled "The Faith That Heals" in the June 18, 1910, issue of *The British Medical Journal*. This article, prompted by controversy over several high profile claims of faith healing and miraculous cures, proposes that "faith has always been an essential factor in the practice of medicine." He defines faith in broad terms—spirituality, faith in one's fellow human beings, and faith in one's self—all of which can contribute to the healing process. Osler suggests that rather than rejecting claims of faith healing out of hand, such claims should be brought under the microscope of medicine to be studied.

> *Others will analyze [faith's] workings, the relation to suggestion, to the subconscious self, etc. Not a psychologist but an ordinary physician concerned in making strong the weak in mind and body, the whole subject is of intense interest to me. I feel that our attitude as a profession should not be hostile . . . A group of active, earnest, capable young men are at work on the problem, which is of their generation and for them to solve. The angel of Bethesda is at the pool—it behooves us to jump in!*

His words are equally as applicable in the context of modern medicine at the dawn of the twenty-first century as they were at the dawn of the twentieth century. And in the words of another great scientist, Albert Einstein:

> *A legitimate conflict between science and religion cannot exist . . . science without religion is lame, religion without science is blind.*

The Pastoral Care Department at The Johns Hopkins Hospital continues to carry on a tradition of spiritual care begun in years past with the Visiting Clergy Service. The first full-time paid director was Reverend Harry Price (1956–1963), a Methodist minister who also happened to be the husband of the Vice President of Nursing at that time. Both had been part of the Army's 118th General Hospital, a Hopkins medical unit during World War II.

Following Reverend Price came the long and capable tenure of Reverend Clyde Shallenberger (1963–1993), a Church of the Brethren minister who also provided leadership in the creation of the hospital's Ethics Committee and Consultation Service. I have over-seen the department since 1994. A Presbyterian minister, I have worked to establish a pastoral education program for clergy and lay volunteers and assisted in providing education about spirituality and healing to the medical, nursing, and allied healthcare professionals throughout The Johns Hopkins Hospital, as well as through the Hopkins Schools of Medicine and Nursing. Each spring the chaplain's office sponsors a multidisciplinary Institute on Spirituality and Medicine that examines different clinical areas in the context of spirituality. The education program is also clinically oriented, providing for hundreds of supervised hours of clinical training and a nine-month residency program.

The department owes most of its success to its staff chaplains, support staff, chaplain interns and residents, and many volunteer adjunct chaplains of diverse religious traditions who have shared their lives and talents with the patients, families, and staff members of The Johns Hopkins Hospital over the years.

To understand the importance of the hospital chaplain, it may be necessary to deal first with the common stereotypes of chaplains and clergy often seen in the media. With the rare exception of characters like Father Mulcahy in the television series *M*A*S*H,* clergy have frequently been typecast as either pious fops or malevolent hypocrites. In the very rare instances when hospital chaplains were pictured, it was inevitably at the bedside of a dying patient. (As a side note, I once had a small role as a Catholic priest in a short-lived series in the mid-1980s called *Buck James*, starring Dennis Weaver, based on the life of a trauma surgeon at the hospital where I was working as a chaplain. In a show that supposedly prided itself on accurate portrayals of hospital life, I found myself arguing that Catholic priests hadn't mumbled Latin liturgies since 1963, during the second Vatican Council, when it was decreed that the Mass should be spoken in the vernacular of the people. And, yes, I was only seen at the bedside of a dying patient.) Needless to say, with these popular stereotypes prevalent in the media, my first visit with hospital patients who have had little previous contact with hospital chaplains inevitably start off with the patient saying, "Chaplain, my doctor didn't tell me I was *that* sick!"

A professional certified healthcare chaplain must meet a number of educational and training requirements. The person in this position has been ordained in a recognized faith community, endorsed by that community for ministry as a chaplain, earned at least a bachelor's degree and in addition had three years of graduate theological education (often a master's degree), and put in at least 1,600 supervised hours of clinical pastoral education. The hallmarks of clinical pastoral education include integration of theology and the behavioral sciences, and the ability to correctly assess and provide appropriate spiritual care in an interfaith and pluralistic context.

At Hopkins, and other hospitals, the primary role of the professional chaplain is to correctly identify patients' spiritual needs and resources, while carefully respecting each individual's religious or spiritual orientation. We take care not to infringe upon a patient's religious rights through proselytizing or otherwise violating a patient's religious or spiritual beliefs, rituals, customs, or practices.

With our specialized training and orientation, the staff and I make it our mission to assess and understand the religious and spiritual language and world view of the patients we encounter. It is our role to provide spiritual care and support appropriate to the patient's clinical and spiritual context, including emotional and spiritual support for patients who may view themselves as agnostic or atheist. Then, when appropriate, our professional connection to the religious community allows us either to provide or facilitate sacramental ministries, liturgies, rituals, customs, or practices requested by patients and to provide some liaison and education between the religious community and the healthcare environment. It is our hope that in providing these services, we enhance the healing that occurs at this hospital and help patients and their loved ones with the difficult struggles they often face at times of medical crisis.

—The Reverend Stephen Mann,
M.Div., B.C.C.
Director, Pastoral Care
The Johns Hopkins Hospital
March 10, 2000

APPENDIX

Prayers of Hope, Consolation, and Thanksgiving

As you have read in the preceding stories, prayer is a powerful force in the lives of many people at times of medical crisis and, of course, at many other times of life. Following is a sampling of prayers of different sorts—traditional prayers that have been used through the ages, passages from the Bible and Koran, prayers from Johns Hopkins chaplains, from clerics of different faiths and denominations, and the personal prayers of patients and their loved ones left at the statue of The Divine Healer at The Johns Hopkins Hospital. These personal prayers are quoted here anonymously to protect the privacy of the writers.

Prayers of Hope

> *Then the eyes of the blind will be opened, and the ears of the deaf will be unstopped. Then the lame will leap like deer, and the tongue of the dumb will one day shout for joy.*
>
> —ISAIAH 35:5–6

> *I am the Lord that healeth thee.*
>
> —EXODUS 15:26

Appendix

God, the sun has not yet pushed back the darkness of the night—but we know that it will for it has been so ever since the dawn of time.

And so it is with our fears and our concerns as the time for surgery, with all its attendant mysteries, approaches. Those anxieties are pushed back as we recognize that we are in Your presence, for there is nowhere that we can be where You are not. I pray for Dr. [name] and for all those who will assist him/her in [patient]'s surgery and postoperative care. Give them keen minds and swift but compassionate hands as they become the instruments of Your healing.

To those of us who wait the seeming endless hours until surgery is complete, the assurance is that we, too, are surrounded by Your presence and embraced by Your love. AMEN.

—JOHNS HOPKINS CHAPLAIN EMERITUS CLYDE R. SHALLENBERGER FOR

A PATIENT BEFORE EARLY SURGERY

May the One who blessed our ancestors—
Sarah, Rebecca, Rachel, and Leah,
Abraham, Isaac, and Jacob,
bless and heal the one who is ill:
[name], daughter/son of [name].
May the Holy One, the fountain of blessings,
shower abundant mercies upon her/him,
fulfilling her dreams of healing,
strengthening her with the power of life.
Merciful One:
restore her,
heal her,
strengthen her,
enliven her.
Send her complete healing
from the heavenly realms,
a healing of body and

a healing of soul,
together with all who are ill,
soon, speedily, without delays;
and let us say:
Amen!

—*MISHABERACH*, TRADITIONAL JEWISH PRAYER FOR THE SICK

O God, the source of all health: So fill my heart with faith in
Your love, that with calm expectancy I may make room for Your
power to possess me, and gracefully accept Your healing; through
Jesus Christ our Lord. Amen.

—EPISCOPAL BOOK OF COMMON PRAYER

Ah, happily do we live in good health among the ailing; amidst
the ailing we dwell in good health.

—BUDDHIST PRAYER

Do not fear for I am with you, do not be afraid for I am your God:
I will strengthen you, I will help you, I will uphold you with My
victorious right hand.

—ISAIAH 41:10

By Your power, great God, our Lord Jesus Christ healed the sick
and gave new hope to the hopeless. Though we cannot command or
possess Your power, we pray for those who want to be healed.
Mend their wounds, soothe fevered brows, and make broken spirits whole again. Help us to welcome every healing as a sign that,
though death is against us, You are for us, and have promised renewed and risen life in Jesus Christ our Lord.

—PRESBYTERIAN BOOK OF COMMON WORSHIP, PASTORAL EDITION

O Father of mercies and God of all comfort, our only help in time
of need: We humbly beseech Thee to behold, visit, and relieve
Thy sick servant [name] for whom our prayers are desired. Look

Appendix

upon him/her with the eyes of thy mercy; comfort him with a sense of Thy goodness; preserve him from the temptations of the enemy; and give him patience under his affliction. In Thy good time, restore him to health, and enable him to lead the residue of his life in Thy fear, and to Thy glory; and grant that he may dwell with Thee in life everlasting; through Jesus Christ our Lord. Amen.

—EPISCOPAL BOOK OF COMMON PRAYER

Let me not pray to be sheltered from dangers,
but to be fearless in facing them.
Let me not beg for the stilling of my pain,
but for the heart to conquer it.
Let me not crave in anxious fear to be saved,
but for the patience to win my freedom.

—BUDDHIST PRAYER

Lord Jesus Christ, Good Shepherd of the sheep, You gather the lambs in Your arms and carry them in Your bosom: We commend to Your loving care this child [name]. Relieve his/her pain, guard him from all danger, restore to him Your gifts of gladness and strength, and raise him up to a life of service to You. Hear us, we pray, for Your dear name's sake. Amen.

—EPISCOPAL BOOK OF COMMON PRAYER

Hey God, it's me, the big pain. Try and help me get over what I'm going through. Teach me to forgive, give me the will to help my-self and others. You are the only one who can help me right now.

—ANONYMOUS

Thus saith the Lord, the God of David thy father, I have heard thy prayer, I have seen thy tears; behold, I will heal thee.

—2 KINGS 20:5

Appendix

Say unto them O Muhammad: For those who believe it is a guidance and a healing.

—KORAN 41:44–51

Blessed Lord, we ask Your loving care and protection for those who are sick in body, mind, or spirit and who desire our prayers. Take from them all fears and help them put their trust in You, that they may feel Your strong arms around them. Touch them with Your renewing love, that they may know wholeness in You and glorify Your name, through Jesus Christ our Lord.

—OCCASIONAL SERVICES, A COMPANION TO

LUTHERAN BOOK OF WORSHIP

And when I am sick, then He restores me to health.

—KORAN 26:80

I will also heal the blind and the leper, and bring to life the dead, by leave of Allah.

—KORAN 3:49

For He hath not despised nor abhorred the affliction of the afflicted; neither hath He hid His face from him; but when he cried unto Him, He heard.

—PSALMS 22:24

Dear God, I ask for healing of body, mind, spirit for my sister through this time during and after her surgery. Guide and lead the doctors and nurses through this period for her peace of mind for myself and family.

—ANONYMOUS

Dear God. Please take care of Joe. He really needs Your help.

—ANONYMOUS

Appendix

Dear Heavenly Father, be with Tom. Bless him and heal him so that his quality of life returns. In Jesus' Name, Amen.

—ANONYMOUS

Merciful God, Your healing power is everywhere about us. Strengthen those who work among the sick; give them courage and confidence in everything they do. Encourage them when their efforts seem futile or when death prevails. Increase their trust in Your power even to overcome death and pain and crying. May they be thankful for every sign of health You give, and humble before the mystery of Your healing grace; through Jesus Christ our Lord.

—PRESBYTERIAN BOOK OF COMMON WORSHIP, PASTORAL EDITION

God, don't let my daddy die.

—ANONYMOUS CHILD

Dear God. Please heal Joy's body of cancer. Be with her and her family. Give us strength.

—ANONYMOUS

Great multitudes followed [Jesus], and He healed them all.

—MATTHEW 12:15

Is there any sick among you? Let him call for the elders of the church; and let them pray over him, anointing him with oil in the name of the Lord. And the prayer of faith shall save the sick, and the Lord shall raise him up; and if he have committed sins, they shall be forgiven him.

—JAMES 5:14–15

Lord Jesus Christ, You chose to share our human nature, to redeem all people, and to heal the sick. Look with compassion upon Your servant whom we have anointed in Your name with this holy oil for the healing of body and spirit. Support him/her with Your power, comfort her with Your protection, and give her the strength to fight against evil. Since You have given Your servant a share in Your own passion, help her to find hope in suffering, for You are Lord forever and ever.

—THE ROMAN [CATHOLIC] RITUAL, PASTORAL CARE OF THE SICK

And when Jesus was come into Peter's house, He saw his wife's mother laid, and sick of a fever. And He touched her hand, and the fever left her; and she arose, and ministered unto them.

—MATTHEW 8:14–15

And heal the sick that are therein, and say unto them, The kingdom of God is come nigh unto you.

—LUKE 10:9

Arise, go thy way: thy faith hath made thee whole.

—LUKE 17:19

Heal me, O Lord, and I will be healed; save me and I will be saved, for Thou art my praise.

—JEREMIAH 17:14

By stretching forth Thine hand to heal; and that signs and wonders may be done by the name of Thy holy child Jesus.

—ACTS 4:30

God of compassion, you have given us Jesus Christ, the great physician, who made the broken whole and healed the sick. Touch our wounds, relieve our hurts, and restore us to wholeness of life, through the same Jesus Christ our Lord.

—PRESBYTERIAN BOOK OF COMMON WORSHIP, PASTORAL EDITION

Appendix

Almighty God, we pray that our brothers and sisters may be comforted in their suffering and made whole. When they are afraid, give them courage; when they feel weak, grant them Your strength; when they are afflicted, afford them patience; when they are lost, offer them hope; when they are alone, move us to their side. In the name of Jesus Christ, we pray.

—THE UNITED METHODIST BOOK OF WORSHIP

Please watch over Bill's eyes today.

—ANONYMOUS

Dear God, Just let her know You are with her.

—ANONYMOUS

Dear Lord, Reggi is in need of Your holy help. Please lend Your helping hand and bring his strength up to fight this horrible infection. Thank You!

—ANONYMOUS

Dear Father in Heaven, please make a way for me and my child.

—ANONYMOUS

We have waited four months and driven fifteen hours to the number one hospital in America, to see the number one ophthalmologist in America. And he can't tell us what's wrong, much less be able to fix it. Lord, You are the great physician, You are the Lord, our Healer. Father, You are now our only hope. No one else can help us. Father, You are mighty and righteous, faithful and true. We have put our trust in You, Lord. Reach Your hand down and touch her, heal her, Father, for You are the only one who can.

—ANONYMOUS

And when He was come into the house, the blind men came to Him: and Jesus saith unto them, Believe ye that I am able to do this? They said unto Him, Yea, Lord. Then touched He their eyes, saying, According to your faith be it unto you. And their eyes were opened.

—MATTHEW 9:28–30

God of love, ever caring, ever strong, stand by us in our time of need. Watch over this child who is sick, look after him/her in every danger, and grant this child healing and peace. We ask this in the name of Jesus the Lord.

—THE ROMAN [CATHOLIC] RITUAL, PASTORAL CARE OF THE SICK

But for you who fear My name, the sun of righteousness will rise with healing in its wings; and you will go forth and skip about like calves from the stall.

—MALACHI 4:2

And Jesus went about all Galilee, teaching in their synagogues, and preaching the gospel of the kingdom, and healing all manner of sickness and all manner of disease among the people.

—MATTHEW 4:23

Father, in the name of Jesus, I come to You asking that Your light shines through me all day, and Your presence is around me every day. Give me brand new mercies to help me endure all my situation, and fill me with Your love. In Jesus' name I pray to You. Amen.

—ANONYMOUS

I lay my hands upon you in the Name of our Lord and Savior Jesus Christ, beseeching Him to uphold you and fill you with His grace, that you may know the healing power of His love. Amen.

—EPISCOPAL BOOK OF COMMON PRAYER

Almighty God, source of human knowledge and skill: Guide physicians and nurses and all those You have called to practice the arts of healing. Strengthen them by Your life-giving Spirit, that, by their ministries, the health of people may be promoted and Your creation may be glorified. Through Jesus Christ our Lord.

—OCCASIONAL SERVICES, A COMPANION TO

LUTHERAN BOOK OF WORSHIP

Prayers of Consolation

Yea, though I walk through the valley of the shadow of death, I will fear no evil: for Thou art with me; Thy rod and Thy staff they comfort me.

—PSALMS 23:4

O God, we have experienced a torrent of emotions tonight. We are reminded of the excitement and the anticipation at the birth of a child—the despair that came with the news of that child's illness—the pain and anguish, the anger and bewilderment over why a child should have to experience such suffering—those times when we wondered if You had abandoned us—the frustration when there seemed to be no answers to our prayers.

Your word reminds us that there is a time to be born and a time to die. And so there is—but that dying never seems to come at the right time, whatever the "right time" is. We can never forget what has been experienced in the death of a loved child. Grant that we may find strength in the awareness that You will never leave us or forsake us.

May Your peace be eternally on those children we remember tonight—and may some of that same peace be upon each of us as well. AMEN.

—JOHNS HOPKINS CHAPLAIN EMERITUS CLYDE R. SHALLENBERGER,

TRIBUTE SERVICE FOR CHILDREN WHO DIED AT THE

JOHNS HOPKINS HOSPITAL

Appendix

Please, God, no more painful days like today.

—ANONYMOUS

My two boys are in Your hand, Lord Jesus.

—ANONYMOUS

Blessed be the God and Father of our Lord Jesus Christ, the Father of mercies and the God of all consolation, Who consoles us in all our affliction, so that we may be able to console those who are in any affliction with the consolation with which we ourselves are consoled by God. For just as the sufferings of Christ are abundant for us, so also our consolation is abundant through Christ.

—2 CORINTHIANS 1:3–5

Lord Jesus Christ, we come to You sharing the suffering that You endured. Grant us patience during this time, that as we live with pain, disappointment, and frustration, we may realize that suffering is a part of life, a part of life that You know intimately. . . . Renew us in our spirits, even when our bodies are not being renewed, that we might be ever prepared to dwell in Your eternal home, through our faith in You, Lord Jesus, who died and are alive for evermore. Amen.

—THE UNITED METHODIST BOOK OF WORSHIP

Father, may all who suffer pain, illness, or disease realize that they have been chosen to be saints and know that they are joined to Christ in His suffering for the salvation of the world. We ask this through Christ our Lord.

—THE ROMAN [CATHOLIC] RITUAL, PASTORAL CARE OF THE SICK

Dear Lord, You have provided so much that is wondrous. I don't want to overlook the wonders of life. This prayer is for me and others who are in pain and grief. Bless those we love and guide

Appendix

them safely. Bring the light and wisdom to us all so we can guide each other in Your name.

—ANONYMOUS

Dear God, I have never asked for anything, but now I need the strength to be able to handle things. Please help my wife overcome this illness. Please! Help me.

—ANONYMOUS

Almighty and everlasting God, comfort of the sad and strength to those who suffer: Let the prayers of Your children who are in any trouble rise to You. To everyone in distress, grant mercy, grant relief, grant refreshment, through Jesus Christ our Lord.

—OCCASIONAL SERVICES, A COMPANION TO
LUTHERAN BOOK OF WORSHIP

Lord, this teenage son is riding my last nerve because he doesn't tell the truth and is extremely lazy. Please help us. Amen.

—ANONYMOUS

Lord, help all parents of children on alcohol and drugs.

—ANONYMOUS

Merciful God, enfold this child in the arms of Your love. Comfort these parents in their anxiety. Deliver them from despair and give them patience to endure and guide them to choose wisely for their child, in the name of Him who welcomed little children, Jesus Christ our Lord.

—PRESBYTERIAN BOOK OF COMMON WORSHIP, PASTORAL EDITION

Lord Jesus Christ, by Your patience in suffering You hallowed earthly pain and gave us the example of obedience to Your Father's will: Be near me in my time of weakness and pain; sustain *me by Your grace, that my strength and courage may not fail; heal me according to Your will; and help me always to believe that what happens to me here is of little account if You hold me in eternal life, my Lord and my God. Amen.*

—EPISCOPAL BOOK OF COMMON PRAYER

Have mercy upon me O Lord; for I am weak; O Lord, heal me; for my bones are vexed.

—PSALMS 6:2

Please take care of my grandpa who went to live with You September 14th. Watch over him and keep him safe. Amen.

—ANONYMOUS (AGE 8)

Dear Jesus, Please help my husband. Help him so he won't suffer. Please work a miracle and cure his pancreatic cancer. He is too young to die. Thy will be done.

—ANONYMOUS

Dear Lord or Whomever Above, People say You move in mysterious ways. Then why have You given my mother cancer again? She tells me to have faith in You, to believe in You . . . How can I have any faith? Enough of the testing.

—ANONYMOUS

Almighty God, shield of the oppressed, hear us as we pray for the friendless and the lonely, the tempted and the unbelieving. Be merciful to those who suffer, in body or in mind, to those who are in danger or distress, and who have suffered loss. Let Your love surround the infirm and aged. Be especially near to those who are passing through the valley of death. May they find eternal rest and light at evening time; through Jesus Christ our Lord.

—THE UNITED METHODIST BOOK OF WORSHIP

Appendix

My all powerful God, help me remember that You have a plan for my life and that's all I need to know.

—ANONYMOUS

Magnified and sanctified be the name of God throughout the world which He has created according to His will. May He establish His kingdom during the days of your life and during the life of all of the house of Israel, speedily and soon; and say ye, Amen.

May His great name be blessed forever and ever.

Blessed and praised, glorified and exalted, extolled and honored, adored and lauded be the name of the Holy One, blessed be He, whose glory transcends, yea is beyond all praises, hymns and blessings that man can render unto Him; and say ye, Amen.

May there be abundant peace from heaven, and life for us and for all Israel; and say ye, Amen.

May He who establishes peace in the heavens, grant peace unto us and unto all Israel; and say ye, Amen.

—KADDISH, JEWISH MEMORIAL PRAYER FOR THE DEAD

Prayers of Thanks

Blessed are You, HaShem, our God, King of the Universe, Who formed man with intelligence, and created within him many openings and many hollow spaces; it is revealed and known before the Seat of Your Honor, that if one of these would be opened or if one of these would be sealed it would be impossible to survive and to stand before You (even for one hour). Blessed are You, HaShem, Who heals all flesh and does wonders.

—ASHER YATZAR, JEWISH DAILY PRAYER

Dear Allah, I owe You, for such nice medical school around, in our times. Thank You very much.

—ANONYMOUS

Appendix

Dear Jesus,

Thank You for making my grandmother-in-law feel better. I am so glad You heard my prayers. Please make her even more better so she can come home for Christmas.

I love You so much.

—ANONYMOUS

Daughter, Thy faith has made you well.

—MARK 5:34

Dear God, Thank You so very much for watching over my baby angel through her surgery and recovery. And thank You for bestowing the knowledge and compassion to the doctors and nurses who continue to care for her. Amen.

—ANONYMOUS

I come here to stand beneath Your statue, and to give thanks and praise to You and Your Father for the third anniversary of my son's surgery and healing performed by Your faithful servant Dr. Benjamin Carson. To God be all Glory for His mercy. I love You, Lord, and will ever kneel before You in praise.

—ANONYMOUS

Thank You, Lord, for giving me this day.

—ANONYMOUS HOSPITAL EMPLOYEE

Thank You for people.

—ANONYMOUS CHILD

Thank You, God, for this miracle today. I saw my grandson walk to me. I'm thankful for all You've given him.

—ANONYMOUS

Appendix

Dear Jesus, I thank You for healing my body with my whole heart. You are the head of my life and You are the head of this blessed hospital. Everyone who enters is under Your Almighty High Power. Bless this hospital, its doctors, nurses, and all support team members as well as the rest of the entire staff. Again, dear Lord—thanks.

—ANONYMOUS

Dear Lord & Savior. Thank You for Your many blessings. Mom is undergoing a procedure involving her bile duct and liver and pancreas region. Please make her healthy!

—ANONYMOUS

Dear God, Thank You for blessing us with this new liver. Help me to get even better!

—ANONYMOUS

Hello, Jesus. Help my daughter wake up, please. Keep her from being frightened. Thank You for this day!

—ANONYMOUS

The peace of the sculpture is the peace we all seek everywhere and ever more. Thank You.

—ANONYMOUS

Dear God—Once again I am here by the statue—it is so inspirational. Thank You for hearing and answering my prayers. Please continue to keep watch over us and help us to stay strong in our recovery.

—ANONYMOUS